Praise for

THE EATING DISORDER ......

"*The Eating Disorder Trap* is an excellent guide for understanding the complexities of eating disorders. I recommend it as a valuable resource for healthcare professionals, as well as for those who find themselves or their loved ones in this trap."

—Anita Johnston, PhD
Author of *Eating in the Light of the Moon*

"Emerging from Robyn Goldberg's extensive clinical history treating countless clients, this book offers families, individuals, and clinicians a thoughtful overview of the entire spectrum of eating disorders. I appreciate her weight-inclusive approach and wise recommendations."

—Jennifer L. Gaudiani, MD, CEDS-S, FAED
Author of *Sick Enough*
Founder and Medical Director of Gaudiani Clinic

"*The Eating Disorder Trap* is an essential resource. It respects those suffering and equips those who can come alongside and support recovery in an empowering context of informed compassion. Not just a must-read—a must-use."

—Nancy L. King, MS, RDN
Coauthor of *Moving Away from Diets*
Founder and Director of Your Life Nutrition

"I foresee this book becoming the groundwork for an eating disorder clinician's foundation along with supervision. Robyn helps us understand that recovery is not the client or clinician's burden, but rather a collective cultural issue that must be challenged in order to support eating disorder recovery for all bodies. This book is inclusive of all genders and fat positive. This is *the* book for any healthcare provider in training who may not necessarily specialize in eating disorders. It has the power to help future providers have a basic healing infrastructure to help people get the care they need. It's the change our culture so desperately needs."

—Julie Duffy Dillon, MS, RDN, NCC, CEDRD-S
Host of *The Love Food Podcast*

"Robyn Goldberg is a master at cultivating true healing from an eating disorder, and this skill feels like her gift to the world. *The Eating Disorder Trap* will help you turn down the voice of the eating disorder and step fully into your own."

—August McLaughlin
Author of *Girl Boner*
Host and Creator of Girl Boner Radio

"*The Eating Disorder Trap* is a timely publication, coming as it does as a stand-alone piece packed full of wisdom, research, and a sensitive respect for professionals and families in the trenches to win the battle against a deadly enemy that has invaded their lives. Robyn has left no stone unturned, using non-shaming vocabulary for gender and body size and shape."

—Adrienne Ressler, LMSW, CEDS, F.iaedp
Vice President – Professional Development
of the Renfrew Center Foundation

"*The Eating Disorder Trap* is a call to action for all professionals. It raises awareness for any reader, especially those in a position to recognize eating disorders in a timely fashion. Robyn busts many myths."

—Ovidio Bermudez, MD, FAAP, FSAHM, FAED, F.iaedp, CEDS
Chief Clinical Education Officer at the Eating Recovery Center

"Robyn Goldberg offers a clear and comprehensive picture of how eating disorders emerge and the challenges in treating them. I recommend this book as a starting point and framework for thinking about how dietitians such as myself can develop a better means for meeting the nutritional needs of people in recovery from all types of eating disorders."

—Ralph E. Carson, RD, CEDRD, PhD
Author of *The Brain Fix*
Senior Clinical and Research Advisor
at the Eating Recovery Center

"Comprehensive, orderly, and backed by years of solid experience, Robyn Goldberg's *The Eating Disorder Trap* is your go-to for the facts on eating disorders!"

—Kathryn Cortese, LCSW, ACSW, CEDS
Editor-in-Chief of the Gurze/Salucore
Eating Disorders Resource Catalogue

"This book offers something for everyone. Whether you are someone suffering from an eating disorder, a family member or friend of a sufferer, clinician, coach, or teacher, you will find yourself flipping through this book to garner insights on a regular basis."

—Reba Sloan, MPH, LRD, FAED
Fellow of the Academy for Eating Disorders

"Start here! *The Eating Disorder Trap* will help those with eating disorders, their loved ones, and clinicians new to the field find their path toward healing and helping."

—Leslie Schilling, RDN, CEDRD-S
Creator and Coauthor of *Born to Eat*
Nutrition Therapist

"This is one of the best books I have read in some time. As an expert therapist in the field of eating disorders, *The Eating Disorder Trap* will be in my office as a standard read for consulting professionals, patients, and family members."

—James D. Runyan, MS, LMFT, LPC, CEDS, F.iaedp
Past President of the IAEDP

"Everyone needs to read this book. *The Eating Disorder Trap* is modern, progressive, and eloquently debunks the myths we have about eating disorders. Whether you need a strong starting place, or you are looking to advance your existing knowledge, Robyn's guide is for you."

—Signe Darpinian, LMFT, CEDS-S
Coauthor of *No Weigh!*
President of the SF Bay Area IAEDP Chapter

"The Eating Disorder Trap will not only benefit those with eating disorders, but the hundreds of millions of individuals known as 'disordered eaters.' Robyn Goldberg offers a compassionate, intelligent road map through the morass of finding one's way out, toward freedom."

—Francie White, PhD, RDN
Tending the Feminine Psyche—Eating Disorder
Professional Trainings

"The Eating Disorder Trap is a rich resource of both researched knowledge and clinical wisdom about the assessment and treatment of eating disorders. Robyn translates complicated clinical and medical information into accessible and practical recommendations."

—Douglas W. Bunnell, PhD, CEDS-S
Fellow of the Academy for Eating Disorders

"The eating disorder field has needed this book for a long time. Robyn dismantles nutrition myths and stresses that an 'empathetic collaboration' between providers, clients, and family is essential to recovery. Essential read for providers and loved ones."

—Stephanie Brooks, MS, RDN, CEDRD-S
Founder of Bay Area Nutrition, LLC

"Robyn Goldberg does an excellent job of presenting complex issues associated with eating disorders in a way that is informative and easy to understand. I would highly recommend *The Eating Disorder Trap* for anyone who wants to expand their eating disorder knowledge."

—Lesley Williams, MD, CEDS
Author of *Free to Be Me*

"This long-overdue book supports both professionals and loved ones with the facts about eating disorders and how to best support those affected by them."

—Anna M. Lutz, MPH, RDN, CEDRD-S
Owner of Lutz Alexander Nutrition Therapy

"I love Robyn Goldberg's passion in *The Eating Disorder Trap*. The reader can tell she has extensive eating disorder experience, compassion for patients, and a desire to help build a supportive environment to guide their recovery. I highly recommend this book."
—Kathy King, RDN, LD, FAND
CEO of Helm Publishing, Inc.

"Robyn Goldberg provides a savvy, to-the-point review of eating disorders and their nutritional effects. I am grateful to have a resource to provide to clinicians who may not work often with eating disorder clients."
—Jill Sechi, MS, RD, CEDRD-S

"Virtually every person with an eating disorder has been harmed in an unintentional way by a health professional or 'expert' who did not know what they were doing. Robyn Goldberg's *The Eating Disorder Trap* is a much-needed set of makeup lessons."
—Michael P. Levine, PhD, FAED
Fellow of the Academy for Eating Disorders
Emeritus Professor of Psychology at Kenyon College

"*The Eating Disorder Trap* is a wonderful how-to guide for clinicians and loved ones! It's full of helpful content that will equip clinicians and loved ones with the tools to best support individuals in recovery. I *highly* recommend this book!"
—Jennifer Rollin, MSW, LCSW-C
Founder of the Eating Disorder Center

"In a Westernized society ridden with such a prolific diet culture, *The Eating Disorder Trap* is a *must-read*! In succinct and simple language, Robyn offers the reader a clear description and understanding of eating disorders and best practices in treatment as well."
—Michele Lob PsyD, MFT, CEDS
DBT Center of Orange County

"The reader is in for a much-needed new look at the complicated subject of eating disorders. Created to speak to coaches, teachers, and those new to the field, even a seasoned expert will appreciate this as a review. *The Eating Disorder Trap* should be the go-to for easy-to-understand medical, psychological, and nutritional information."

—Pamela Kelle, RDN, CEDRD

"This thorough, comprehensive book is a *must-read* for coaches, teachers, or anyone working with teenagers and adults who wants to better understand the complex nature of eating disorders and how best to deal with those who struggle with this insidious disease."

—Leslie Kaplan, MD
Adolescent and Young Adult Medicine

"A must-read for healthcare providers supporting clients or patients with eating disorders. Even after thirty-one years of practice, I find this as my go-to resource for client interview questions, statistics for my lectures, and targeted explanations about the psychological and physiological side effects of eating disorders."

—Diana Lipson-Burge, RDN, CEDRD

"*The Eating Disorder Trap* is a brilliant addition to the books in the current field of eating disorders highlighting anorexia nervosa and bulimia nervosa. The nutrition chapters are a standout and will be a wonderful resource for years to come."

—Melainie Rogers, MS, RDN, CDN, CEDRD-S
Founder and CEO of Balance Treatment Center

THE
EATING
DISORDER
TRAP

ROBYN L. GOLDBERG, RDN, CEDRD-S

Foreword by Carolyn Costin, MA, Med., MFT, CEDS, FAED

THE EATING DISORDER TRAP

A Guide for Clinicians and Loved Ones

BOOKLOGIX˙
Alpharetta, GA

The information provided in this book is not intended to be used for purposes as medical treatment and instead of seeing your eating disorder–registered dietitian, physician, mental health provider, and other providers.

ISBN: 978-1-63183-776-0 - Paperback
eISBN: 978-1-63183-777-7 - ePub
eISBN: 978-1-63183-778-4 - mobi

Library of Congress Control Number: 2020903008

Printed in the United States of America   1 1 2 4 2 0

∞This paper meets the requirements of ANSI/NISO Z39.48-1992 (Permanence of Paper)

Cover illustration and design by Tracie Crowser
Illustrations by Austin Baechle
Author photo by Michael Roud

Health at Every Size® is a registered trademark of the Association for Size Diversity and Health (2011).

This book is dedicated to all of the clinicians and loved ones who are striving to help and support someone they know with an eating disorder.

One cannot think well, love well, sleep well, if one has not dined well.

—Virginia Woolf

CONTENTS

FOREWORD

Today there are many books on the market about eating disorders. How does one choose? Robyn L. Goldberg, RDN, CEDRD-S, has given readers a new option, offering a comprehensive summary that describes how to better understand "the eating disorder trap." Robyn has taken her years of experience as a dietitian treating eating disorders and come up with a succinct overview of the myriad of questions posed by her clients and their family members. Through writing this book, Robyn provides information she has gleaned from her experience that can also help clinicians and other treatment providers better comprehend and help clients with the often difficult road of recovery.

Robyn's book covers the basic diagnostic criteria and medical symptoms of eating disorders in a simple-to-read format. Even more importantly, Robyn helps readers comprehend the mindset of someone trapped in an eating disorder. She describes the concept of how each person with an eating disorder has, over time, developed an eating disorder self, and how those trying to help them need to recognize this concept and work to strengthen the client's underlying healthy self in order for them to recover.

Patients, family members, and treatment providers can all get valuable information from this book. This book covers a lot of material— Robyn delineates how to conduct a nutrition interview, she reviews the specific macronutrients, and she explains common myths and important facts as they relate to eating disorder clients. Robyn weaves in her years of experience, while also adding in the expertise of other colleagues.

The Eating Disorder Trap is an easy-to-digest book that offers a look at important issues that must be dealt with for anyone wanting to understand or help those afflicted with an eating disorder.

—Carolyn Costin, MA, Med., MFT, CEDS, FAED
Founder of the Carolyn Costin Institute
Author of *8 Keys to Recovery from an Eating Disorder* and *The Eating Disorders Sourcebook*

INTRODUCTION

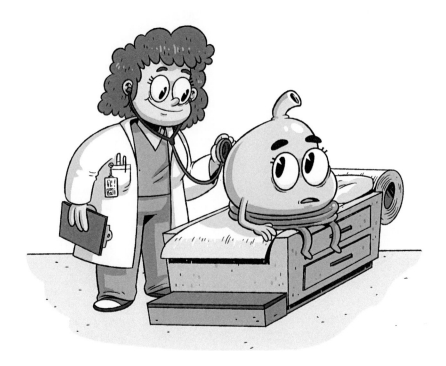

It is estimated that the prevalence of eating disorders has doubled worldwide from 2013–2018 as compared to 2000–2006.[1] People of all ages and genders suffer with these life-threatening disorders.[2] Eating disorders do not discriminate, and it is likely we all have a loved one or a close friend who is quietly struggling with an eating disorder. It is a complicated and challenging battle, rife with guilt, shame, insecurity, and uncertainty. These disorders are usually kept secret, and it is not uncommon for those struggling to be suffering in silence. Even so, statistics reveal the harrowing truth that this epidemic is spreading quicker than ever before.[3]

An eating disorder has a substantial impact on one's ability to experience joy and fulfillment. It decimates friendships and relationships, it derails careers and personal aspirations, it can lead to traumatic medical situations, and in the most serious of cases, it can lead to death. As sufferers literally deprive their bodies of the fruits of life, they fall deeper into the disease, leading them to dire consequences.

Despite their gravity, eating disorders remain largely misunderstood. Even in the "age of information," it is common for there to be assumptions, stigma, stereotypes, and misinformation related to the origin, experience, and treatment of these disorders. It can be difficult for physicians, psychologists, psychiatrists, registered dietitians, and other treatment providers to properly diagnose and treat eating disorders. The longer the eating disorder goes unnoticed and untreated, the more the behaviors flourish in the dark.

The lack of knowledge about eating disorders isn't only evident in the average person. Sadly, while the incidence of eating disorders has steadily increased since 1950,[4] the medical profession has not kept up with this growth. Adolescent medicine remains the only medical specialty that mandates training in eating disorders. Although statistics show that many people develop eating disorders in their teenage or college years, these disorders can occur over the individual's lifetime, and are not limited to adolescence. This, then, can make medical professionals treating adults ill-equipped to provide crucial treatment to a large number of struggling individuals.

Shockingly, the mental health field has also failed to rectify this shortcoming. Even though eating disorders have the second-highest mortality rate (following opioid addiction) of any psychiatric illness, psychiatry programs do not require eating disorder knowledge or training. Only a small number of psychology or counseling programs offer either.[5]

Medical and mental health professionals often have a lack of eating disorder training. The lack of understanding and training on the part of medical and mental health professionals can make the patient's problem worse through perpetuated stigma, judgment, delay in diagnosis, and/or misdiagnosis.

These illnesses are not only dangerous, but also expensive. Much of that expense, however, can be alleviated by early diagnosis and appropriate treatment. As a professional specializing in identifying and treating eating disorders, I have gathered extensive knowledge, training, and experience in this field. Since the fields of medicine, physiology, and neurochemistry are evolving so rapidly, it is no wonder that professionals can hardly stay afloat. My goal with this book is to offer professionals across the health spectrum insight and basic tools to use with their patients. In addition, I have collaborated with many other trained eating disorder professionals, and have utilized their expertise in the development of this book.

The ultimate objective of this book is to bridge the existing gap among professionals, those suffering from an eating disorder, their loved ones, and the public. I hope for this book to serve as a resource for anyone who may encounter eating disorders in their professional or personal life. The recognition and understanding of these disorders can make all the difference. Early intervention is a true game-changer, saving lives and finances, in the combat against these powerful diseases.

This book is intended for anyone who hopes to further their awareness and understanding of eating disorders through practical and implementable tools. This book offers easy-to-understand medical, psychological, and nutritional information. Whether you are a practicing clinician, registered dietitian, school coach, personal trainer, loved one, or someone who is personally struggling with an eating disorder, this book is for you.

Due to the lack of consistent terminology and to make an effort to be inclusive, I have chosen to use the following terminology suggested by Andrew Sage Mendez-McLeish, MEd, EdS, a professor of child development, education, and parenting education at California State University Dominguez Hills and Pasadena City College:

Estrogen-based bodies—typically cisgender women, pre-medical-transition trans men, and nonbinary and/or agender individuals who are assigned female at birth.

Testosterone-based bodies—typically cisgender men, pre-medical-transition trans women, and nonbinary and/or agender individuals who were assigned male at birth.

You will also see the words "obese" and "obesity" written as "ob*se" and "ob*sity."

Although these words are used in medical and health communities, many practitioners in the field recognize that the terms are stigmatizing to those in larger bodies.

Those reading this book are likely a diverse group of talented, intelligent, and caring individuals looking for accurate information about eating disorders. The age-old adage of "know thine enemy" certainly applies here. Awareness and education are key to combating the escalation of eating disorders. Only when we know exactly what we are fighting can we win the battle.

For those who may interact with individuals struggling with an eating disorder, there is immense opportunity for your actions and awareness to enact change and healing. The more clinicians and supporters understand the distinguishing characteristics of eating disorders, the earlier interventions will occur, the fewer complications will arise over time, and the better and quicker the recovery.

In reading this book, you will learn the basics of eating disorders, gain an understanding of the current research and strategies used with this population, learn helpful language to use when communicating with a patient who may be struggling, and become familiarized with screening questions to help identify eating-disordered behavior. This book has been divided into four parts.

In Part I (Chapters 1–3), we will review the types and incidence of eating disorders, and discuss how to best help people who are struggling with an eating disorder. Part II (Chapters 4–7) will cover the more technical aspects of eating disorder assessment, and a breakdown of how each body part is impacted by an eating disorder. Part III (Chapters 8–11) describes the macronutrients: carbohydrates, proteins, fat, and water. And lastly, in Part IV (Chapters 12–13), we discuss the recovery process.

I hope you utilize these skills in your daily practice and contact with patients and loved ones. It cannot be emphasized enough that knowledge can help you avoid disasters. Your knowledge may be the key in helping someone transform a confusing and dark path into one of awareness, self-understanding, security, and self-acceptance. And, of course, this knowledge will add value to your professional practice, and possibly, your own life.

Collaboration amongst the various disciplines—medical, nutrition, and psychotherapy—is key. Getting everyone on the same page is a requirement for creating a meaningful and effective treatment program for those struggling with an eating disorder. Professional team members may have different philosophies, approaches, personalities, and expertise. Each member, though, is responsible for adjusting the mix to ensure the right balance is found so that a positive difference is made in the lives of patients.

I hope this book will impress upon you the importance of clinicians in all disciplines working together as a team to combat these disorders. You will also walk away with a better understanding of who is to be part of the team. Clinicians do not need to stand alone in treating these formidable illnesses. In fact, treatment is more effective when it involves a comprehensive team of trained eating disorder professionals. This collaboration could be crucial in effecting change in how eating disorders are diagnosed and treated.

The expert contributors and I have a combined experience greater than ten decades. This includes experience in working directly with individuals with eating disorders, advocacy work, presenting at national and international conferences, acting as resources for local and national publications, and being resources for the media on pressing issues in the eating disorder community. Over these decades, we have been in the trenches combating these disorders from all sides, and have gained a fair amount of insight and experience doing so. My interest in this field has led me to read hundreds of articles and a multitude of books related to eating disorders. In doing so, I have found that much of what I am presenting in this book is missing from other books on the market on the subject of eating disorders.

Through offering in-depth insight and information, this book takes on the medical, nutritional, physical, and psychological components of eating disorders. This will then propel professionals to make correct diagnoses and provide appropriate treatment. Gaining and implementing this knowledge is key to combating eating disorders from all sides, and to reversing the concerning trend of the last fifty years. I want to combine the insight and diverse experiences that I have had, and offer practitioners a path to becoming more well-rounded and informed professionals. For our nonprofessional readers, I want you to have a more comprehensive understanding of these complex illnesses. In this way, you will know what medical, nutritional, and psychological concerns professionals should be addressing should you need their services.

My greatest hope is that anyone who reads this book walks away feeling empowered and emboldened to fight eating disorders—either for their own recovery, or for the recovery of a loved one, a client, or a patient.

Introduction Notes

1. M. Galmiche et al., "Prevalence of eating disorders over the 2000–2018 period: a systematic literature review," *American Journal of Clinical Nutrition* 109, no. 5 (May 2019): 1402–1413.

2. Keski-Rahkonen, Wade, and Hudson, in M. Tsuang and M. Tohen (eds.), *Textbook in Psychiatric Epidemiology* 3rd ed. (Chichester, England: John Wiley & Sons, Ltd., 2011).

3. K. Johnson et al., "Eating Disorders: The Weight of Food," *US Pharmacist* 38, no. 9 (2013).

4. J. Hudson et al., "The prevalence and correlates of eating disorders in the National Comorbidity Survey Replication," *Biological Psychiatry* 61, no. 3 (February 2007): 348–358.

5. T. Insel, "Post by Former NIMH Director Thomas Insel: Spotlight on Eating Disorders," National Institute of Mental Health, February 24, 2012.

PART I

GET TO KNOW ED:
THE INCIDENCE OF EATING DISORDERS

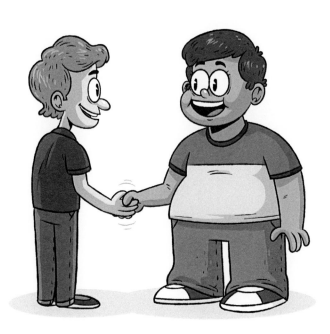

CHAPTER 1

WHAT YOU NEED TO KNOW: NAMING THE PROBLEM

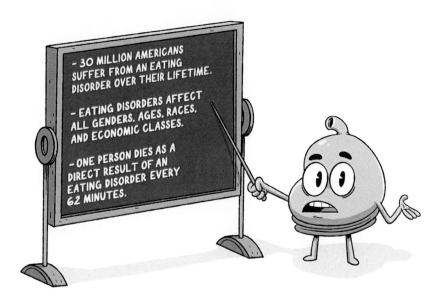

- 30 MILLION AMERICANS SUFFER FROM AN EATING DISORDER OVER THEIR LIFETIME.

- EATING DISORDERS AFFECT ALL GENDERS, AGES, RACES, AND ECONOMIC CLASSES.

- ONE PERSON DIES AS A DIRECT RESULT OF AN EATING DISORDER EVERY 62 MINUTES.

STATISTICS PROVIDED BY EATING DISORDERS COALITION.

It would be a grave understatement to refer to eating disorders as the silent epidemic. Daily, we see people affected with eating disorders like anorexia nervosa, bulimia nervosa, and binge-eating disorder. Yet just a small percentage of those affected actually come forward, admit they have an illness, and seek treatment for their condition. As active members of the eating disorder community, we often witness firsthand the tragic consequences of clients' behaviors being dismissed or unnoticed by clinicians, coaches, dentists, or other healthcare professionals who do not have a working knowledge of eating disorders.

All too often, a lack of training and education in eating disorders leads to incidences of missed or erroneous diagnoses. This can lead to the alienation of struggling patients, and to insufficient or improper interventions. For example, gynecologists may be unaware that missed periods can be a warning sign of malnutrition, and dentists may attribute dental erosion to acid reflux without considering bulimia nervosa as a cause. Many opportunities at intervention are missed due to insufficient awareness. These missed opportunities lead to real-life implications of worsening symptoms, prolonging of eating disorder behaviors, deteriorating health, and sometimes even to lives lost. This book's aim is to help save lives by improving diagnostic acumen and treatment recommendations. Knowledge is power. Unawareness can cause errors, and we need to combat it with education, understanding, and empathy.

Awareness includes knowing the stigma that can go hand in hand with eating disorders, and doing one's best to use language that is not judgmental. This helps clients not feel alienated. There is only a small window of opportunity for getting through to clients, helping them feel supported and understood, and engaging them in treatment. This window shuts very quickly if the patient feels judged or unheard.

These oversights are often unintentional. No physician (or other healthcare provider) wants to hurt their patients. Their Hippocratic oath would not allow it. Like many others, these professionals have not received the proper training to know how to communicate with the eating disorder patients they many encounter. As a result, they may make statements that cause patients to feel judged, persecuted, or misunderstood.

One such oversight is when an untrained clinician suggests a patient lose weight. The quest for thinness in our society, promoted by diet culture, has engrained damaging messages into the minds of clinicians and laypeople alike. Diet culture disguises itself under words like "health" or "wellness." The problem is there is a very narrow margin diet culture uses to define what constitutes health or wellness. Clinicians who have internalized the values of diet culture can make suggestions that will further hurt a person with an eating disorder.

It can be intimidating to have a client with a diagnosis that is unfamiliar to you. Having taken the oath to "do no harm," medical professionals often appropriately refer clients out whom they feel they lack the skills and expertise to treat. As well-intentioned as this may be, this may thrust patients with eating disorders into "medical no-man's-land"—the primary care physician may believe it is a job for the psychiatrist, and the psychiatrist may believe the eating disorder is an issue for the primary care physician to treat. This can lead to a series of referrals as the patient's disorder continues to worsen. Feelings of rejection and alienation can increase, and the patient's faith in being able to get appropriate help, and their motivation to recover, can decrease. Having patients who rarely feel comfortable being transparent and asking for help doesn't make things any easier. Their eating issues may have been dismissed by parents, coaches, or medical professionals. They may have been praised for their weight loss. Conversely, they may have been shamed about their weight by peers, family members, and doctors, and being a victim of weight stigma, have a harder time coming forward for help.

Ultimately, of course, comprehensive treatment requires a multidisciplinary team. A multidisciplinary team would ideally include a primary care physician, a registered dietitian, a mental health provider, and a psychiatrist if needed. Sometimes the team can also include a meal companion, nurse practitioner, and family therapist.

The Statistics Are in . . . They Are Concerning

While doctors and clinicians may be busy bouncing the ball back and forth coming up with few meaningful solutions, patients could be dying. About thirty million Americans of all ages and genders suffer from an eating disorder. These numbers are growing, and hospitalization rates for eating disorder patients have increased 18 percent between 1999 and 2001.[1, 2]

Due to the pervasiveness of diet culture, our society places significant value on how we look. Appearance seems to be everything. We are inundated with marketing that promises diet culture will bring us love, fulfillment, and happiness. We are told these coveted results will be had as long as we eat, exercise, dress, pluck, wax, and spend money the "right" way. With all of the societal pressure to fit a certain "ideal," it is no wonder, then, that so many individuals have complicated relationships with food, exercise, and body image. The emphasis on external appearances can be a huge contributor to eating-disordered behaviors. In fact, many individuals do not realize they are engaging in behaviors that may be concerning. Things like restricting calories or compensating for calories consumed are seen in our culture as positive "lifestyle changes." Unfortunately the changes that usually occur are the development of unhealthy ideals and behaviors. One out of four people who chronically diet will develop a full-blown eating disorder.[3]

The most concerning and prevalent eating disorders that negatively impact our society are outlined below. This is not a complete list of all the eating disorders.

Anorexia Nervosa

Anorexia nervosa, the first eating disorder to be recognized in the Diagnostic and Statistical Manual of Mental Disorders (DSM), is characterized by restriction of food intake leading to weight loss, difficulty maintaining appropriate body weight for height and age, and distorted body image. Individuals struggling with anorexia nervosa often have an altered perception of how their bodies look, as well as a crippling fear of gaining weight or becoming "fat." This is the disorder that most people commonly think of when they think of an eating disorder. It is the third most common chronic disease among young people ages fifteen to twenty-four (0.3–0.4 percent of young cisgender women and 0.1 percent of cisgender men are suffering from it at any given time). Some people believe individuals with anorexia nervosa "just want to be thin" and, therefore, simply need to eat more. The reality is these individuals are experiencing severe struggles and have ten times the risk of dying compared to their same-aged peers. These tragic statistics make it unsurprising that anorexia nervosa has the highest mortality rate of any mental illness.[4]

Bulimia Nervosa

Bulimia nervosa is also a formidable disorder characterized by a cycle of binge-eating followed by compensatory behaviors (vomiting, laxative use, excessive exercise, fasting, diuretic or other medication use) to obtain relief from uncomfortable feelings, uncomfortable levels of fullness, and/or not being able to sit with eating a particular food or food group. Results published in *Biological Psychiatry* have found that 1.5 percent of cisgender women and 0.5 percent of cisgender men will struggle with bulimia nervosa during their lifetime.[5]

Binge-Eating Disorder

Binge-eating disorder is a newer diagnosis that is no less serious, ranking as the most common eating disorder in the United States among adults. It is three times more common than anorexia nervosa and bulimia nervosa combined, and more common than breast cancer, HIV, and schizophrenia. A shocking 3.5 percent of cisgender women and 2 percent of cisgender men will develop binge-eating disorder.[6]

Other Specified Feeding or Eating Disorder (OSFED)

OSFED includes individuals who do not meet the full criteria for the other eating disorders. Some examples of OSFED are:

Atypical Anorexia Nervosa—people who restrict as in anorexia nervosa, yet may be in higher-weight bodies. That they are in higher-weight bodies can make this diagnosis further stigmatizing.

Pica—eating non-nutritive substances in place of food.

Other eating behaviors considered disordered, but not included in the DSM, are:

Diabulimia—manipulating prescribed insulin to promote weight loss.

Exercise Bulimia—using exercise to "purge" calories.

Orthorexia—eating exclusively "clean" or "healthy" foods, leading to malnutrition.

People with OSFED have the same medical risks as people with the other eating disorders. However, they may appear unaffected. These disorders can happen to anyone, regardless of age, race, culture, gender, or ethnicity. Individuals who identify as transgender experience eating disorders at rates significantly higher than cisgender individuals.

Cisgender men have a higher rate of mortality from eating disorders than cisgender women, and while people of color have similar rates of eating disorders, they are significantly less likely to receive help for their eating issues.[7]

These disorders do not occur in a vacuum. Many who suffer from an eating disorder also struggle with other mental illnesses, such as depression and anxiety, substance use, post-traumatic stress disorder, and obsessive-compulsive disorder. Each comorbidity amplifies the destructive effect of the other.

Despite the prevalence and severity of these life-threatening diseases, only a very small percentage of those struggling with an eating disorder receive treatment.

Even the Professionals Need Help

How does this happen? This is because most healthcare clinicians are simply not required to undergo eating disorder education or training. At the core, the problem is a lack of education. Most psychotherapists receive minimal and basic exposure to eating disorders. Adult, child, and adolescent psychiatrists have no mandated eating disorder training in their residency requirements. If elective rotations in eating disorders are offered, most residents do not take advantage of them. Adolescent medicine historically has been the only medical specialty that mandates eating disorder training.

The ideal situation would be for eating disorder training to become mandatory for all healthcare providers. Such training should address the professional's own relationship with food, movement, weight, body image, and belief system around diet culture. Healthcare providers can use a weight-inclusive approach, while rejecting and not idealizing specific body shapes and sizes. I wrote this book because I did not want to wait for such necessary changes to be mandated and enforced. I do not want individuals with eating disorders to fall through the cracks.

Where Do We Go from Here?

Just like with any other illness, early detection of eating disorders is crucial in tackling the problem head on and preventing it from worsening. The longer a patient struggles with an eating disorder, the harder it is to break the cycle. It is a deep-seeded illness, and one that can impact the root of a patient's very existence. Catching an eating disorder early is similar to treating cancer in its beginning stages. The consequences of not doing so can be equally severe. The more the eating disorder becomes engrained in an individual's life, the more significantly it alters their mind and body.

While many view eating as a recreational activity and a deserved pleasure, for some, it is seen as a scary experience and far from enjoyable. At the end of the day, our bodies need food for sustenance and survival. To illustrate this, let us use a car as an example. Regardless of how shiny it is on the outside, a car will not serve its primary function if it does not have gasoline in the tank to make it go. Our bodies are the same; food is the fuel. Food allows our legs to carry us through the day, allows our arms to hug those we love, and allows our brains to communicate our essence to the world around us.

When we fail to put gas in the tank, or food in our body, those primary functions stop working. Starvation leads to malnutrition, which is a global assault to the body. All organs are affected—the kidneys, heart, skin, brain, gastrointestinal tract, teeth, hair, and virtually every other organ system of the body. Failing to recognize the signs and symptoms of an eating disorder, healthcare professionals can put an individual in grave danger. It may take full-blown heart failure or other major organ damage before the pieces are put together.

The effects of the eating disorder worsen the longer the disorder is left untreated. As time goes by, it may no longer be a single organ system that needs to be treated, but rather four, five, or six systems or ailments that have to be addressed. Treatment becomes more complex and expensive, and individuals may become unable to pay for needed medical care.

Eating disorders also impact fundamental brain activity. A healthy person, for example, is able to recognize hunger and how it impacts them: lethargy, irritability, and maybe even slower cognitive abilities. Individuals with eating disorders also experience these symptoms, but through regular conditioning, may have lost their recognition of hunger.

The solution here is clear: catching eating disorders early in their development leads to earlier treatment that leads to earlier recovery. If we nip a disorder in the bud before symptoms worsen, the behaviors do not have the opportunity to become engrained. As clinicians, we have the ability, obligation, and opportunity to acquire eating disorder knowledge and awareness. This knowledge will enable early intervention and ultimately save lives.

Chapter 1 Notes

1. Y. Zhao and W. Encinosa, *Hospitalizations for Eating Disorders from 1999 to 2006*, HCUP Statistical Brief 70 (Rockville, MD: Agency for Healthcare Research and Quality, April 2009).

2. J. Hudson et al., "The prevalence and correlates of eating disorders in the National Comorbidity Survey Replication," *Biological Psychiatry* 61, no. 3 (February 2007): 348–358.

3. G. C. Patton et al., "Onset of adolescent eating disorders: population based cohort study over 3 years," *British Medical Journal* 318, no. 7,186 (March 1999): 765–768.

4. J. Arcelus et al., "Mortality rates in patients with anorexia nervosa and other eating disorders. A meta-analysis of 36 studies," *Archives of General Psychiatry* 68, no. 7 (July 2011): 724–731.

5. J. Hudson et al., "Prevalence and correlates of eating disorders."

6. "Statistics & Research on Eating Disorders," National Eating Disorders Association, accessed December 20, 2019, www.nationaleatingdisorders.org/statistics-research-eating-disorders.

7. "Statistics & Research on Eating Disorders," National Eating Disorders Association.

CHAPTER 2

CAN WE TALK?
MAXIMIZING YOUR TIME
WITH THOSE STRUGGLING
WITH AN EATING DISORDER

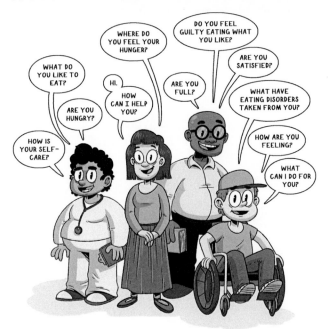

We need to talk.

It is not you, it is us. All of us.

In the first chapter of this book, I offered a general overview of eating disorders, as well as the supporting statistics to demonstrate how serious and prevalent these diseases are within our society.

Eating disorders are not rare. I truly believe anyone would benefit from gaining a working knowledge of eating disorders. The reality is, if you do not run into people with eating disorders in your career, you likely will in your personal life. Eating disorders impact about twenty million cisgender women and ten million cisgender men in the United States alone.[1] A survey of approximately three hundred thousand college students found that transgender college students had over four times greater risk of being diagnosed with anorexia nervosa or bulimia nervosa, and two times greater risk of eating disorder symptoms such as purging compared to their cisgender female peers.[2,3] Regardless of age, gender, race, and sexual orientation, your child, your family member, your colleague, your boss, your neighbor, and your friend could all be affected and at risk.

Therefore, I urge all of you to familiarize yourself with the symptoms of eating disorders, and educate yourselves, so that you will be able to help people in need. In writing this chapter, I had in mind the primary professionals who usually come across this patient population—physicians, dietitians, and therapists. However, this information is also invaluable for dentists, physical therapists, personal trainers, coaches, educators, school counselors, religious leaders, family members, and friends. What category do you fall under? And how can you help? Contemplating the following questions is a great place to start.

How Much Time Do I Spend with People?

If you are a teacher, school principal, coach, or school nurse, think about how much time you spend with the students each day. It is likely that you spend more time with your students than you do with your own family members. For about eight hours a day and five days a week, you witness their mealtimes, social interactions, mood, and appearance. This probably makes you privy to more information than the parents, who may just see them for a few hours in the evening and on weekends. This puts you in a great position to notice any concerning signs or covert calls for help.

The same situation can hold true for others, whether they be trainers, religious leaders, or other helping professionals. Adults who live alone may only see their family members once every few months on holidays. Yet they may see their trainer several times a week, or attend religious services weekly. If one has their eyes open, these regular interactions can reveal concerning behaviors.

If your profession is one that involves being a regular fixture in another individual's life, you are a person of trust who has the opportunity to witness potential eating disorder signs or symptoms.

What Information Am I Learning about People?

Doctors, therapists, or registered dietitians are likely not spending large chunks of time with their patients or clients on a daily basis; however, the time they do spend with them is meaningful, telling, and one of high intensity.

Therapists often ask clients to share their deepest emotional struggles and vulnerabilities and process them in order to overcome them.

Doctors examine the individual's physical body in a way that untrained family or friends cannot. They have the opportunity to ask questions, assess well-being, and screen for health concerns with tests and other measurements.

The insight gained in these encounters is more telling than other ordinary encounters. This then places the clinician in a vital position for intervention. Prompt intervention at the earliest sign of an eating disorder is ideal. Is there significant weight loss? This is especially suspicious for an eating disorder when seen in children, adolescents, and young adults. Other causes of significant weight loss (such as cancer or diabetes) are usually easily discernible and are less common than eating disorders.[4, 5, 6]

Below are five simple questions that can be used as a screening tool to assess for need for a referral to an eating disorder specialist:

1. Do you have a poor relationship with food?
2. Do you feel guilty after eating certain foods?
3. Do you frequently compensate for eating too much or for eating a "forbidden" food?
4. Do you have a history of chronic dieting?
5. How much of the day do you spend thinking about food, eating, or your weight?

These questions are easy to ask even if you feel you have insufficient training or time to address them. The initial screening does not necessarily mean the one asking will be the one offering the formal assessment or treatment. Its prime purpose is to determine if a referral for an in-depth assessment would be beneficial. The Academy for Eating Disorders[7] and the National Eating Disorders Association[8] websites are just two of the many online resources that will help a provider find a local eating disorder specialist.

Unfortunately, even glaring signs of eating disorders are often ignored. This oversight can be deadly. It is estimated that there is an average span of five years between the time of the first visit to the doctor and the time the diagnosis of an eating disorder is made. Also worrisome is that it could take months or years before treatment actually starts.

Meet Rae, a Dancer Who Thought They Were Not Small Enough

This is an example of a teenager I will call Rae, who struggled with anorexia nervosa.

The dance teacher notices Rae has lost a significant amount of weight quickly, and asks if there is something wrong. Rae admits that they want to be thin like the other dancers, so they have stopped eating very much. Rae's dance teacher voices her concerns to Rae's parents.

Rae's parents take them to the doctor. The doctor notes that Rae has had weight fluctuations since their last appointment, sensitivity to cold, dry skin, brittle hair, a low heart rate, mood changes, trouble sleeping, and complaints of fatigue. Recognizing these signs as worrisome, the doctor orders labs and refers Rae to a therapist.

Rae's therapist finds that, in addition to their physical symptoms, Rae speaks about food and their relationship to their body in a troubling way. They have a lot of shame and guilt with eating, and feels they still need to lose more weight. Rae's therapist acknowledges that she is well-educated but not well-trained in eating disorders and refers Rae to an eating disorder specialist.

The specialist finds Rae to be in need of a higher level of care, and facilitates getting Rae into an eating disorder–treatment program.

Rae's treatment team consists of a therapist, medical doctor, psychiatrist, and a dietitian. Rae receives the coordinated care they need to process the mental, emotional, and physical deterioration caused by their eating disorder. Rae's parents are also involved with the treatment team. They are updated on Rae's progress and goals, and are asked to attend family meetings.

Rae restores their weight, and is discharged from the eating disorder program. They have been connected to an outpatient treatment team, who will continue to support Rae through their healing process.

Consider the many instances in the above scenario where Rae could have fallen through the cracks. The dance teacher could have ignored or even validated Rae's weight loss, praising them for becoming thinner. The doctor could have just asked the family to come back in six months, and not referred Rae to a therapist. The therapist could have continued seeing Rae despite her lack of experience with eating disorders. The treatment center could have discharged Rae without coordinating care with an outpatient team.

The network of support created among these individuals worked well because they each had a working knowledge of eating disorders, and a desire to help Rae in the best way possible. That one person in Rae's life spoke up about a concerning behavior she noticed, leading to the domino effect of Rae's disorder being detected earlier. This allowed for Rae to receive the comprehensive care they needed to recover, before their disordered behaviors became engrained.

Beginning this domino effect is sometimes as simple as asking the question, "What is going on?" This can be particularly pivotal early on, when the eating disorder behaviors aren't as entrenched in the individual's identity. A simple "What is wrong?" can give them the exact opportunity they have been looking for to admit they are in trouble, scared, confused, and need support.

Yet it is not always that easy. Eating disorders, by nature, are secretive. If you are examining a patient and ask about a potential disordered behavior or symptom, there is always the chance they will flat out lie or completely deny they have an issue. Even when working with a client with an admitted eating disorder, they may simply refuse to engage and you may reach a roadblock where things just "are not working."

Have You Identified Someone Who May Need Help? What Is the Next Step?

First and foremost, lead with compassion. These individuals are struggling with a mental illness that has hijacked their mind, body, and soul. They don't mean for their lies to hurt you; they are not being obstinate when they refuse to get help. They are simply clinging to a coping mechanism that they have found to be their best source of comfort at this time.

As professionals, we sometimes have to approach the individual like a puzzle box, attempting to reach them in varied ways until they open up or become interested in receiving help. If the direct question of "What is wrong?" does not work, try asking the following questions, which give the individual more power and agency:

- What are your goals for working with me?
- What needs can I help you fulfill?
- What are things that are important to you in your life?
- What can I do that would be helpful for you?

It can also help to ask indirect questions about their disorder or their behaviors, such as:

- If weight wasn't a concern for you, would you continue to eat in the way you are eating?
- What do you like to eat, not just what you have been told not to eat?
- Are you worried I may take away the only thing that has helped you feel better about yourself?

Imagine you have struggled with an eating disorder for a while. You have tried all sorts of treatments and coping skills, and you have been to more appointments and clinicians than you can count. Is it likely, then, that you may feel as hopeless and burned out as some of your clients or patients do? Reaching someone who has completely shut themselves down to help is not easy, but it may help to start with what went wrong in their previous experiences. Finding out what didn't work in past encounters can help you move forward with your work. Some sample questions to ask in this regard are:

- What has worked for you in the past, and what has not?
- At what point did you feel things stopped working?
- Where do you think your therapist/treatment team went wrong?

These questions can also be helpful if you feel your treatment has come to a halt. You may have inadvertently said or done something that shut your client down. Being open and honest about what did not work for them can help repair any damage, improve the individual's view about treatment, and help treatment progress forward.

It is important to consider how your messages come across. Sometimes you have the right intentions, yet deliver the message in a way that turns the client off. For example, you may be excited to recommend they vacation in a city you visited on bicycle. If the client has any exercise resistance, or physical limitations, this may come across as insensitive.

Here are some of the best tips I can offer to help you communicate your messages more effectively:

Watch your language (both your body language and your words). Let your body show that you are interested and concerned. Show such expressions in your face, and with your tone. Be mindful of the words you choose and how they may be perceived. Be especially careful with language you use when addressing the body, appearance, food, and movement. Our society is permeated with diet culture language; it is important to ensure the things we say do not reinforce it. It is imperative to be nonjudgmental in discussions about appearance, exercise, and food. Conveying judgment in our statements can be harmful for anyone, but is particularly destructive to someone who struggles with an eating disorder.

Avoid self-disclosure. Yes, it is important that your clients and patients see you as human. After all, no one wants to be treated by a robot they do not know or understand. However, in these circumstances, disclosing about your own eating or movement habits can sometimes cause more harm than good. The meeting is about them, not you. You might accidentally mention a restrictive behavior that to you seems harmless, but to someone with an eating disorder, generates another insecurity or "food rule." How an individual nourishes and fuels themselves is as unique to them as their bodies and their personalities; therefore, disclosing your own practices may not serve anyone and may promote comparison. In instances where the clinician has recovered from their own eating disorder, discretion can be practiced with regard to self-disclosure. In such cases, self-disclosure may actually be validating for the client.

Their body is not your business. Too many people make the mistake of believing a certain body weight, size, or shape is indicative of health, or lack thereof. Comments like, "You do not look like you have an eating disorder," "You do not look so bad," "You do need to lose some weight," or "You should exercise more," are incredibly destructive. They send the message that people with eating disorders need to look a certain way, and people who are "healthy" must look a certain way too.

The discussion of someone's body size, weight, or shape needs to be approached very carefully. When showing concern about potential eating-disordered behavior, discuss the behavior rather than appearances. For example, "I have noticed you have been eating less," or "I am worried that you stay in the bathroom for a while after every meal." Comments that involve assessment of appearance can be triggering for clients. For example, parents who see their loved one and say, "You look so much healthier," or "Wow, they fattened you up in no time," can be causing significant damage to treatment progress.

Do not envy their eating disorder. It is shocking that this even needs to be said. There are horrifying stories of clinicians telling patients, "I wish I had a little bit of what you have," or "I think I would lose weight if I did that," or "I understand why you do that, because I have to exercise a lot to get rid of this belly."

Eating disorders are incredibly traumatizing disorders that can lead to severe health problems and death. They are not something to be desired.

Do not push restriction. Patients are often told to "cut out carbs" or "cut down on dairy." Encouraging restriction can amplify the problems of patients who struggle with an eating disorder.

A former client told me the first time she purged was in response to her doctor telling her to cut more fat out of her diet. At that time, she had already been restricting and had cut everything she could think of out of her diet. So the only remaining option became purging. Having a working knowledge of eating disorders could have helped prevent this; the doctor would have known to not make triggering suggestions.

Set the Example

Becoming aware of the language used in your clients' environment can be a powerful way for you to support your client. Often, friends or family members are unaware of how their words or actions can impact their loved one. They may act as "food pushers," for example, simply trying to help their loved one feel better by offering them food. Or they may be routinely making positive comments about their loved one's appearance. All these actions are well-intentioned but misguided, and should be gently corrected.

Raising awareness about how such remarks affect your client will teach family members or friends how to better support the client. Pushing food can teach the client the habit of comforting emotions with food, even when not hungry. Commenting on appearances may make the client feel pressured to always look a certain way.

Helping individuals with eating disorders involves some learning as well as some unlearning. You will need to learn how to recognize the signs and symptoms of eating disorders, and how to best approach someone who may be struggling. You will need to "unlearn" language that diet culture has engrained in you and learn to speak in a way that deemphasizes body weight, size, shape, and appearance. Focus on the inner beauty of the person, their value system, and how recovery will bring out the best in them.

It is important to acknowledge the shortcomings of our training. Knowing a little about eating disorders does not make you qualified to treat them. As in Rae's story, the therapist knew her limitations and referred Rae to someone who specialized in eating disorders. Take the ego out of the game. It is important to remember that we are all in this together to help the client. If we cannot treat them, the best way to help them is to find someone who can.

If you make the decision to refer this person to a therapist, eating disorder specialist, or treatment program, please do your due diligence first. Do not simply surf the web for treatment programs, but rather look for programs and clinicians who do not promote any form of restriction, dieting, or weight loss. There can be unclear messages when looking for a provider or program, and oftentimes they are disguised as an eating disorder–treatment program. Look for eating disorder–treatment programs that utilize a well-rounded team of professionals: therapists, doctors, psychiatrists, and dietitians.

The old saying "Sticks and stones can break my bones, but words cannot harm me" does not apply to eating disorders. In many cases, it is the words of others that instigate an eating disorder. The right words can be a powerful tool in opening the gates of communication with someone struggling with an eating disorder so healing can start. A meaningful interview process by a professional can make all the difference. I'll discuss that in the next chapter.

Chapter 2 Notes

1. "Statistics & Research on Eating Disorders," National Eating Disorders Association, accessed December 20, 2019, www.nationaleatingdisorders.org/statistics-research-eating-disorders.

2. "Statistics & Research on Eating Disorders," National Eating Disorders Association.

3. E. W. Diemer et al., "Gender Identity, Sexual Orientation, and Eating-Related Pathology in a National Sample of College Students," *Journal of Adolescent Health* 57, no. 2 (August 2015): 144–149.

4. E. Shinohara et al., "Esophageal cancer in a young woman with bulimia nervosa: a case report," *Journal of Medical Case Reports* 1, no. 160 (November 2007): 1–4.

5. F. Navab et al., "Bulimia nervosa complicated by Barrett's esophagus and esophageal cancer," *Gastrointestinal Endoscopy* 44, no. 4 (October 1996): 492–494.

6. S. Amiel et al., "Ketone lowers hormone responses to hypoglycaemia: evidence for acute cerebral utilization of a non-glucose fuel," *Clinical Science* 81 (August 1991): 189–194.

7. Academy for Eating Disorders, www.aedweb.org.

8. National Eating Disorders Association, www.nationaleatingdisorders.org.

CHAPTER 3

IDENTITY CRISIS AND THE DIAGNOSIS OF AN EATING DISORDER: WHO CAN HELP YOU?

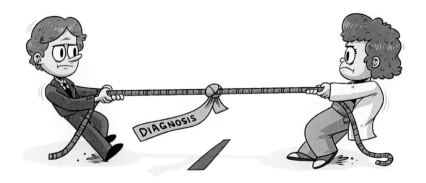

It is a scenario that is all too often played out in the eating disorder realm. The person with an eating disorder and their loved ones do not know who to turn to for help. They may have consulted with medical doctors who were untrained in eating disorders, and uncomfortable with the psycho-social aspects of the eating disorder. They were told their eating disorder is behavioral. "Go to a therapist," is a directive they often hear.

The patient makes an appointment with a mental health clinician. This provider, however, has no training in eating disorders. They are not informed regarding specific screening questions to ask, or how to counsel the individual. Being uncomfortable with the medical aspects of the eating disorder, the mental health provider tells the patient their eating disorder is medical. "Go see your doctor," they direct the client to do.

The patient is now stuck in medical no-man's-land, while desperately trying to find help and support to combat this potentially deadly disorder. As providers and insurance companies battle back and forth about the semantics of their disorder, wanting to leave it in a neat package on the other's doorstep, the patient is left without appropriate care and with increasing feelings of shame and helplessness.

Where can they go? Who can they turn to? It seems like an endless game of finger-pointing, while the patient is left suffering. This is what we mean by "identity crisis." Those with eating disorders are often given the runaround. This can be easily prevented by educating more physicians, therapists, and other medical care providers about eating disorders.

The incidence of eating disorders has continued to rise since the 1950s. Currently, thirty million Americans of various races, ages, genders, and socioeconomic status are suffering from an eating disorder. As more people have been impacted, the diagnostic criteria has accordingly evolved.[1, 2] The diagnostic criteria for eating disorders specified in the Diagnostic and Statistical Manual of Mental Disorders changes with every publication.

Despite the rise in the incidence of eating disorders, specialized training in the medical field has not kept up with this trend. Of 637 medical training programs surveyed, 514 reported that they do not offer rotations in the field.[3] To this day, there is only one medical specialty that mandates training in eating disorders. It is not adult psychiatry or even child and adolescent psychiatry, it is solely adolescent medicine that requires this training.

On the flip side of the coin, psychologists and behavioral health specialists may be uncomfortable treating these disorders because of the medical component. A colleague of mine once suggested to me that psychiatry does not want to deal with medical, and medical does not want to deal with psychiatry.

The psychological *and* medical aspects of eating disorders are of absolute importance; one can't consider one and disregard the other. For example, every organ system is affected by the ravages of malnutrition, and if left unchecked, the patient can suffer more gravely from its long-term consequences.

Insurance companies consider eating disorders behavioral health issues, which means medical coverage can be quite limited, and the patient will have to pay out of pocket for eating disorder–specific medical care.

Furthermore, defining eating disorders as "behavioral health issues" makes it difficult for nutrition services offered by a dietitian to be covered by insurance. To help patients obtain insurance reimbursement, it is best to refer to a registered dietitian nutritionist (RDN) who is also a CEDRD (certified eating disorder registered dietitian). This is the highest level of certification in the eating disorder field for dietitians, and helps clients receive insurance reimbursement.

Eating disorders are comprised of both medical and behavioral issues, and labeling them correctly in this way can lead to better insurance coverage and comprehensive treatment.

What's in a Name?

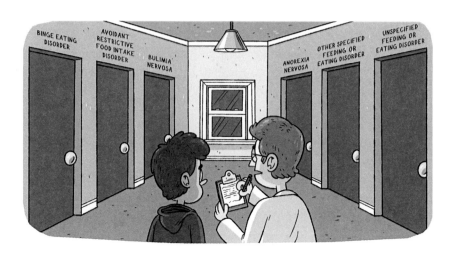

Throughout time, the use of labels, titles, and names have helped us make sense of the world around us. They promote understanding and organization.

The same holds true for diagnostic nomenclature. Over time, certain patterns of behavior and symptoms were grouped together and labeled in an attempt to categorize it all. Similarly, giving diagnostic labels to the different types of eating disorders can help group together their probable causes, potential problem list, and recommended treatment interventions.

In the DSM-5, eating disorders are compiled under the umbrella of "Feeding and Eating Disorders." They are as follows:

Anorexia Nervosa

Anorexia nervosa is the third most common chronic illness among adolescents. The disorder itself is broken down into two categories: restricting type or binge/purge type. According to the DSM-5, anorexia nervosa is the restriction of food which leads to a body weight lower than the individual's natural weight when considering their age, sex, developmental stage, and overall health status.

This disorder is also characterized by an overwhelming fear of "gaining weight" or becoming "fat." The individual also experiences an altered perception of their body and how they actually look. As the malnutrition becomes more severe, and the brain becomes more starved, this altered perception can get worse.

In the Binge Eating/Purging Type of anorexia nervosa (AN-B/P), the individual will "binge" (we will define "binge" in the Bulimia Nervosa section) and then purge. The methods of purging used are the same as those listed in the Bulimia Nervosa section. The other form, Anorexia Nervosa—Restrictive Type (AN-R), involves pure restriction without binges or compensatory behaviors.

Anorexia nervosa has a basis in biological, psychological, and social factors, and is especially linked to issues with control. For example, it is not uncommon for an individual to turn to controlling their food intake (and thus their body shape and size) as compensation for feeling out of control in an area of their life. The comfort they may feel from this false sense of control, however, will do little to help with their life situation, and often leads to even more desire for control and further food restriction.

Bulimia Nervosa

According to the DSM-5, bulimia nervosa involves binging (eating significantly more food than others would normally eat within a short period of time), and then engaging in a compensatory behavior. Compensatory behaviors include self-induced vomiting, laxative use, diuretic use, or compulsively exercising, in an attempt to prevent weight gain. Either one or a combination of these compensatory behaviors can be used, in varying degrees of frequency and severity.

A notable characteristic of this disorder is the lack of control the individual feels when they are binging; they feel unable to stop. It is as if the binge behaviors are controlling them, instead of them controlling their food intake.

Bulimia nervosa behaviors can be triggered by negative body image, a history of trauma, cultural issues, and genetic components.[4, 5] Ironically, bulimia nervosa and binging and purging behaviors can cause weight gain instead of the desired effect of weight loss.

Another trigger can be the common practice of restricting food intake between binge episodes. This deprivation makes it more likely for a binge to occur. The starving brain wants to be fed and will increase our urge to eat, and often eat "more than enough," in case there may be future restriction. While the feeling of guilt for eating so much can be intense, it's important to realize the binge is really an effort to protect the body from starvation.

Binge-Eating Disorder (BED)

Binge-eating disorder is now given its own diagnosis. It was previously placed under the umbrella of Eating Disorder—Not Otherwise Specified (ED-NOS). Binge-eating disorder is similar to bulimia nervosa in that it involves binging. However, binge-eating disorder is different in that the individual does not engage in compensatory behaviors.

The individual with BED often eats when they are not hungry. Because of the shame and humiliation they feel about eating large volumes of food, these individuals usually binge in secret, and when they are alone. These binges happen frequently and the individual feels a lack of control over them, leading to strong negative feelings such as overwhelming guilt, anger, frustration, helplessness, and hopelessness.

BED is the most common eating disorder in adults (60 percent of cisgender women and 40 percent of cisgender men with eating disorders have BED). Binge-eating disorder is three times more common than anorexia nervosa and bulimia nervosa combined.[6] Transgender youth who have experienced higher rates of harassment and discrimination have a higher likelihood of engaging in binge eating, fasting, or vomiting to lose weight.[7]

It is interesting that BED is the eating disorder that is least recognized.[8] This is probably due to the fact that individuals with BED don't often seek help because of the intense shame they feel about their out-of-control eating.

Pica

Pica refers to the persistent eating of nonfood substances that have no nutritional benefit. Examples include eating dirt, clay, chalk, soap, ice, dry paint, or paper. Oftentimes the individual who engages in pica has a mineral deficiency, such as iron.

Rumination Disorder

Rumination is when an individual chews food, swallows it, and either voluntarily or involuntarily regurgitates it. The regurgitated food can be swallowed again, or spit out. Rumination is commonly used as a coping skill when individuals feel uncomfortably full or are experiencing uncomfortable feelings.

Avoidant/Restrictive Food Intake Disorder

Eating issues seen in ARFID can appear in infancy on and lead to severe malnutrition. Unlike anorexia nervosa, however, the food restriction in ARFID has nothing to do with a distorted body image or a desire to change one's weight, size, shape, or appearance. Individuals with ARFID can restrict all food intake or restrict only certain types of food based on texture, color, or smell. A common reason for such restriction is the belief that certain foods will trigger choking or vomiting. The restriction of food choices can get progressively worse, and lead to the same physical consequences as those seen in anorexia nervosa or its variant, atypical anorexia nervosa.

Other Specified Feeding or Eating Disorders (OSFED)

As with BED, OSFED was previously included under the Eating Disorder—Not Otherwise Specified (ED-NOS) category. ED-NOS was a collective term used to identify individuals with a variety of symptoms from the disorders described above who did not meet the full criteria. Historically, individuals labeled with ED-NOS were as likely to die as a result of their eating disorder as individuals with anorexia nervosa or bulimia nervosa.[9]

Some examples of OSFED are:

> **Atypical Anorexia Nervosa**—This diagnosis has most of the same symptoms as anorexia nervosa, but the individual may look "normal" or live in a larger body. An example can be an individual who appears "normal" or lives in a larger body, but who has lost a significant

amount of weight. Because the person does not appear physically malnourished or emaciated, they can fall through the cracks in being diagnosed or with receiving treatment.

Night-Eating Syndrome—This disorder occurs when the individual has difficulty sleeping or struggles to sit with uncomfortable feelings at night and, therefore, wakes up to eat to "medicate" themselves. It is common not to be interested in eating the following morning because of the residual fullness. Many believe that this disorder stems from the individual's belief that eating will help them fall back asleep. It is also likely that not eating enough during the day can drive the nighttime eating. The amount of food eaten during these episodes tends to be less than the amount eaten during binges seen in binge-eating disorder.

Orthorexia—This describes a disorder where individuals limit their intake to only those foods that are deemed "clean" or "healthy." In an effort to have a pristine diet, individuals restrict their food more and more until their intake can become inadequate in every category of protein, carbohydrate, fat, and calories. The focus becomes more and more about what foods one *cannot* eat instead of what foods one *can* eat. It is also common for these individuals to exercise in excess of their body's capability.

Unspecified Feeding or Eating Disorder (UFED)

UFED is the category that includes any eating disorder that does not fit any of the above. This could be a diagnostic code used when a clinician first sees someone with an eating disorder, but has not yet established the exact eating disorder diagnosis.

It is important to note that all of these disorders carry severe risk. It is not uncommon for those with OSFED or UFED to have severe symptoms. Children often present with atypical presentations of eating disorders (called "early onset eating disorders"), but can be already dangerously ill when first seen. One study from Australia done on five-to-thirteen-year-olds showed that 61 percent had life-threatening illness at time of presentation.[10] Even those with binge-eating disorder can develop medical complications unrelated to weight. Examples include trauma and stigma.[11, 12]

Categorizing these behaviors into specific diagnoses is invaluable in their recognition and treatment. It is also important to not allow these labels to monopolize your attention. Many individuals can display symptoms of one disorder, and with time, their behavior may morph into another disorder. For example, someone may present with anorexia nervosa, then develop binging behavior, and end up with bulimia nervosa.

Conversely, we can argue that the label does not matter. I know, I know, it is confusing! We just covered how helpful they are and why we need them. Yet what truly matters when it comes to treatment is the behaviors themselves. It is more important to consider what the behaviors are, how long the individual has been engaging in them, and how severe and frequent they have become. It is these aspects that determine what support and treatment methods are needed.

Furthermore, the individual's motivation for their behaviors needs to be addressed in treatment. Two individuals may meet the criteria for anorexia nervosa, but one may have unconsciously developed it to feel control over an abusive childhood, while the other may have been triggered by an attempt to achieve higher athletic performance. Just as their motivations for disordered eating differ, so will their motivations for recovery, and recognizing this can be critical in providing effective care.

Labels can also become complicated when an individual improves with treatment. For example, someone with bulimia nervosa may stop purging as they progress, but still engage in binging behaviors. Does that mean the diagnosis should change to binge-eating disorder? Changes in the diagnostic type of eating disorder can complicate insurance coverage as well as treatment.

Other psychiatric disorders commonly co-occur alongside the eating disorder. Up to 50 percent of those with an eating disorder will suffer from depression. Fifty-five to sixty-five percent of those with anorexia nervosa also have an anxiety disorder.[13] Alcohol and substance use disorders are four times more common in individuals with eating disorders.[14] At the end of the day, the label alone does not determine the nutritional, psychological, or medical interventions needed; it is important to pay attention to the behaviors as well, and how they may change over time.

Chapter 3 Notes

1. J. Hudson et al., "The prevalence and correlates of eating disorders in the National Comorbidity Survey Replication," *Biological Psychiatry* 61, no. 3 (February 2007): 348–358.

2. D. Le Grange et al., "Eating disorder not otherwise specified presentation in the US population," *International Journal of Eating Disorders* 45, no. 5 (July 2012): 711–718.

3. F. Mahr et al., "A national survey of eating disorder training," *International Journal of Eating Disorders* 48, no. 4 (May 2015): 443–445.

4. D. Inniss et al., "Threshold and subthreshold post-traumatic stress disorder in bulimic patients: prevalences and clinical correlates," *International Journal of Eating and Weight Disorders* 16, no. 1 (March 2011): e30–36.

5. B. S. Dansky et al., "The National Women's Study: relationship of victimization and posttraumatic stress disorder to bulimia nervosa," *International Journal of Eating Disorders* 21, no. 3 (April 1997): 213–228.

6. "Statistics & Research on Eating Disorders," National Eating Disorders Association, accessed December 20, 2019, www.nationaleatingdisorders.org/statistics-research-eating-disorders.

7. R. Watson et al., "Disorder eating behaviors among transgender youth: Probability profiles from risk and protective factors," *International Journal of Eating Disorders* 50, no. 5 (May 2017): 515–522.

8. R. Watson et al., "Disorder eating behaviors among transgender youth."

9. "Statistics & Research on Eating Disorders," National Eating Disorders Association.

10. S. Madden et al., "Burden of eating disorders in 5–13-year-old children in Australia," *The Medical Journal of Australia* 190, no. 8 (April 2009): 410–414.

11. R. Puhl et al., "Obesity stigma: important considerations for public health," *American Journal of Public Health* 100, no. 6 (June 2010): 1019–1028.

12. D. V. Sheehan et al., "The Psychological and Medical Factors Associated with Untreated Binge Eating Disorder," *Primary Care Companion for CNS Disorders* 17, no. 2 (April 2015).

13. "Statistics & Research on Eating Disorders," National Eating Disorders Association.

14. "Statistics & Research on Eating Disorders," National Eating Disorders Association.

PART II

EVALUATION AND ASSESSMENT

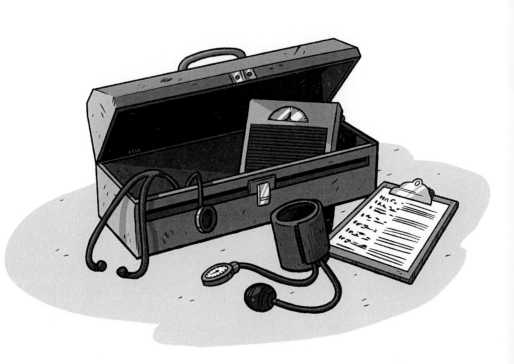

CHAPTER 4

"TRUTH" IN NUMBERS: THE TOOLS AT OUR DISPOSAL

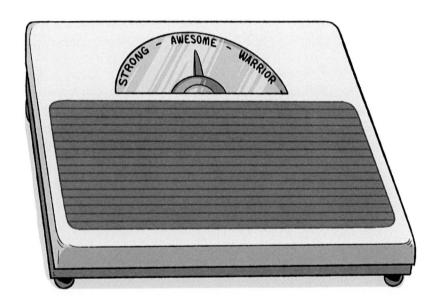

Let's take a moment to discuss a revolutionary concept: numbers, although they have contributed greatly to humankind, are at times completely and utterly arbitrary.

Just like scattered letters on a page, numbers have no meaning on their own. It is only when we group them together, and interpret them, that we give them a meaning. The numbers on a scale that measure your weight are considered a "vital sign," as are your blood pressure, heart rate, and body temperature. Although variations in blood pressure, heart rate, and body temperature can be indicative of ill health, the same does not hold true for weight. Stating a weight is "too high," for example, is completely meaningless. The fact is the charts used to qualify weight (such as the Metropolitan Life Insurance Weight Chart) were put together completely arbitrarily.[1]

Despite the lack of strong evidence supporting such claims,[2, 3] our weight-focused society has hammered into our heads the false belief that having a certain weight or body measurement is directly related to health and personal worth.

This is not right.

Keeping that in mind, we have to ask the question: if numbers qualifying weight were devised completely arbitrarily, is it even possible to define what is "a normal weight"? The simple answer to that question is no!

Let me explain. Every individual has their own "normal weight." This normal weight is achieved when we trust our bodies to eat when we are hungry, eat what we want, and stop when we are full. Trusting our bodies also requires us to be flexible with food—for example, we will nourish ourselves even if we are at a social event or restaurant that doesn't have our preferred foods. Since everyone's hunger level, desired foods, movement, and amount of food to reach fullness is different, it is impossible to label one number or even a range of numbers as "normal."

We are surrounded by weight bias. Clients often experience weight bias from providers in many disciplines, and providers are often unaware that their comments and suggestions are coming from a place of bias. An example is providers who suggest a patient lose weight solely on the basis of the number when the patient is completely healthy. Or providers who suggest patients eat or not eat certain foods, or participate in certain forms of exercise, just based on current diet and exercise trends. Or even providers who suggest patients "just stop overeating," without considering the patient's emotional state or personal history.

To help stop these harmful practices, we need to assist our clients in finding providers who utilize a weight-neutral and weight-inclusive approach. True health promotion happens when clients are not afraid to go to the doctor, because they know they will not be judged for their weight. The following chapters will redefine preconceived definitions of "normal," and demonstrate how normal comes in a variety of shapes and sizes.

Deconstructing BMI

BMI is an arbitrary number that has gained fame in recent years. It is a crude measure of body size in individuals. It is the most commonly used measurement in the medical community to determine health. Millions and millions of people are deemed healthy or not healthy based on this measurement. Despite its widespread use, approximately seventy-five million American adults are misclassified as unhealthy every year.[4]

Standing for Body Mass Index, BMI was created in the nineteenth century by Belgian statistician Adolphe Quetelet. Quetelet initially created the instrument with the intention of using it to measure populations of people, specifically men, not individuals. An entirely different formula was originally used for determining "body size" in cis-female populations, and now doctors use the same equation for all genders. Since the 1970s, the ease of this formula has made it more convenient for healthcare providers, insurance companies, and government statisticians to use it. BMI is much easier to use than more complex measures of body size, such as a skin-fold caliper testing or underwater weight-displacement testing.

The formula is simple; an individual's weight in kilograms is divided by their height in meters squared. Despite the limited parameters used in this formula, nowadays BMI is used to measure and assess complex factors such as body size and medical health.

The general rule is those people who have a BMI of less than 18.5 are considered "underweight," those with a BMI of 18.5 to 25 are considered "normal," those with a BMI of 26 to 29 are "overweight," and those with a BMI of 30 to 39 are considered "ob*se." Anyone with a BMI higher than 40 is considered "morbidly ob*se." Using BMI as a health determinant is very stigmatizing because it places a value on an individual without considering their body composition, personal history, or genetics. Genes determine our biological blueprint, and are important contributors to our body weight, shape, size, appearance, and health.

(The use of the terms "ob*se" and "ob*sity" can be stigmatizing and pathologizing for individuals, hence the use of asterisks.)

Despite not being a medical facility that can make such assessments, many schools now require BMI report cards. Children call these "the fat test" and take on society's faulty understanding that "health" is determined solely by such numbers.

For many reasons, using this oversimplified measurement to generalize overall health is unhelpful and dangerous.

To begin with, BMI does not take body composition into account. Take as an example an athlete who is six foot two and weighs 250 pounds. Their calculated BMI of 32.09 would undoubtedly stamp them as "ob*se." There is no consideration that they are an athlete or body builder, and that much of the 250 pounds is composed of muscle.

BMI doesn't take nutrition into consideration either. An individual may have a BMI of 20.5 and eat dangerously little, but still be labeled "normal." Using this assessment can promote disordered eating, disordered thinking, and an eating disorder.

Measuring BMI involves no evaluative questions. Therefore, we garner no information about energy level, mood, sleep patterns, brain health, or the functioning of hormones. Such information, in contrast to BMI, is incredibly telling of a person's overall health and well-being.

When we consider that BMI only looks at weight and height, it is glaringly obvious that numerous other factors that can determine health are missing. With all these missing factors, using BMI to determine an individual's health status is akin to using a mood ring to diagnose a mental illness. There are too many other elements that need to be considered.

In fact, using weight to determine wellness is ineffective. Weight is nothing more than a measure of gravitational force and should be a neutral term. In space, an NFL lineman who weighs 325 pounds on earth weighs nothing. Their body mass and composition hasn't changed, but their weight has.

There is incredible risk in reducing "health" to such a basic and primitive level. Measures of BMI often cause individuals to become more focused on meeting an "ideal" weight, regardless of the weight being appropriate for their body. It also makes people more likely to focus on dieting and food rules.

BMI also becomes problematic in eating disorder treatment. Insurance companies base their coverage of services on this arbitrary number, without assessing all of the other components involved. Although an individual may be "weight-restored," they may still have unhealthy thoughts about body image, restricting, binging, purging, exercise, and other eating disorder behaviors. Being weight-restored or "within a desirable weight" may not mean that the individual is recovered from their eating disorder.

We are constantly looking for simple and easy assessments of health. BMI, however, is not the answer. With such widespread use, though, you must be wondering: it can't all be negative; there must be some benefit to the use of BMI.

While there are very few benefits to the oversimplified and overgeneralized measurement of BMI, it may be helpful in showing trends. A steep drop or increase in BMI requires further investigation into potential underlying problems.

Overall, the negative impacts of BMI far outweigh the positive. What began as a measurement intended for a limited purpose has become a scientific term twisted into shaming people. BMI assesses health based on very limited information. The Health at Every Size movement is aware of the failings of the BMI, and therefore takes all focus off of weight.

Are There More Useful Tools for Assessing Individuals?

It is clear that BMI measurements are not useful in determining health. They are definitely not useful in assessing for eating disorders. Eating disorders are very difficult to diagnose, especially in the primary care setting. Many clinicians are not familiar with the relatively quick and reliable screening tools available to assess for an eating disorder. Two excellent screening tools are the SCOFF and the EAT-26. The SCOFF was created for the early detection of eating disorders with the hope that early interventions will improve the prognosis for treatment. Unlike other questionnaires that are lengthy and may require a psychologist or specialist to interpret them, the questions of SCOFF were designed to raise suspicion that an eating disorder might exist before rigorous clinical assessment takes place.

SCOFF

- Do you ever make yourself **sick** because you feel uncomfortably full?
- Do you worry you have lost **control** over how much you eat?
- Have you recently lost more than **one stone** (fourteen pounds) in a three-month period?
- Do you believe you are **fat** when others say you are too thin?
- Would you say that **food** dominates your life?

If there are two or more yes answers to the above, there is a very high probability that the client may have anorexia nervosa or bulimia nervosa. Further assessment should be done, or a referral made.

Eating Attitude Test (EAT-26)

An alternative screening tool to the SCOFF is the Eating Attitude Test (EAT-26). This is shown below and can be obtained online at www.eat-26.com. The EAT-26 asks twenty-six questions with answers that are scored. The client answers "Always," "Usually," "Often," "Sometimes," "Rarely," or "Never" to the questions asked. Clearly, the information obtained from the EAT-26 is more comprehensive than the SCOFF. A score greater than twenty warrants further exploration to assess for an eating disorder.

✓ Please choose one response by marking a check to the right of the following statements:	Always	Usually	Often	Some times	Rarely	Never	Score
1. Am terrified about being overweight.	–	–	–	–	–	–	
2. Avoid eating when I am hungry.	–	–	–	–	–	–	
3. Find myself preoccupied with food.	–	–	–	–	–	–	
4. Have gone on eating binges where I feel that I may not be able to stop.	–	–	–	–	–	–	
5. Cut my food into small pieces.	–	–	–	–	–	–	
6. Aware of the calorie content of foods that I eat.	–	–	–	–	–	–	
7. Particularly avoid food with a high carbohydrate content (i.e. bread, rice, potatoes, etc.)	–	–	–	–	–	–	
8. Feel that others would prefer if I ate more.	–	–	–	–	–	–	
9. Vomit after I have eaten.	–	–	–	–	–	–	
10. Feel extremely guilty after eating.	–	–	–	–	–	–	
11. Am preoccupied with a desire to be thinner.	–	–	–	–	–	–	
12. Think about burning up calories when I exercise.	–	–	–	–	–	–	
13. Other people think that I am too thin.	–	–	–	–	–	–	
14. Am preoccupied with the thought of having fat on my body.	–	–	–	–	–	–	
15. Take longer than others to eat my meals.	–	–	–	–	–	–	
16. Avoid foods with sugar in them.	–	–	–	–	–	–	
17. Eat diet foods.	–	–	–	–	–	–	
18. Feel that food controls my life.	–	–	–	–	–	–	
19. Display self-control around food.	–	–	–	–	–	–	
20. Feel that others pressure me to eat.	–	–	–	–	–	–	
21. Give too much time and thought to food.	–	–	–	–	–	–	
22. Feel uncomfortable after eating sweets.	–	–	–	–	–	–	
23. Engage in dieting behavior.	–	–	–	–	–	–	
24. Like my stomach to be empty.	–	–	–	–	–	–	
25. Have the impulse to vomit after meals.	–	–	–	–	–	–	
26. Enjoy trying new rich foods.	–	–	–	–	–	–	
					Total Score =		

Step 1: EAT-26 ITEM SCORING:	
Score each item as indicated below and put score in box to the right of each item	
Items # 1-25:	Item #26 only:
Always = 3	= 0
Usually = 2	= 0
Often = 1	= 0
Sometimes = 0	= 1
Rarely = 0	= 2
Never = 0	= 3

Garner, D. M., Olmsted, M. P., Bohr, Y., and Garfinkel, P. E. "The Eating Attitudes Test: Psychometric features and clinical correlates." *Psychological Medicine* 12, no. 4 (1982): 871–878. Permission for the EAT-26 granted April 9, 2019.

Another evidence-based screening tool is the Eating Disorder

Inventory-3 (EDI-3). This screening takes approximately twenty minutes to administer and twenty minutes to score. The advantage of this screening test is that it assesses for things such as the drive for thinness, body dissatisfaction, and perfectionism. Repeating the EDI-3 over the course of treatment can show trends in the client's progress, which can assist with treatment planning. There is an electronic version of the EDI-3 that scores the test. There is a cost, however, for this electronic tool.

If you are completing the above screening tests for yourself or a loved one, and there is in fact suspicion for the presence of an eating disorder, please alert your healthcare practitioner and ask to be referred to a professional who specializes in the assessment and treatment of eating disorders.

Becoming familiar with and using the different assessment tools discussed will help identify people with eating disorders earlier, and ultimately lead to better outcomes.

Chapter 4 Notes

1. T. Penney et al., "The Health at Every Size Paradigm and Obesity: Missing Empirical Evidence May Help Push the Reframing Obesity Debate Forward," *American Journal of Public Health* 105, no. 5 (May 2015): e38–e42.

2. T. Penney et al., "The Health at Every Size Paradigm."

3. J. Robinson et al., "Health at Every Size: a compassionate, effective approach for helping individuals with weight-related concerns—Part II," *American Association of Occupational Health Nurses* 55, no. 5 (May 2007): 185–192.

4. A. J. Tomiyama et al., "Misclassification of cardiometabolic health when using body mass index categories in NHANES 2005–2012," *International Journal of Obesity* 40, no. 5 (May 2016): 883–886.

CHAPTER 5

WHAT IS NORMAL?
ONE SIZE DOES NOT FIT ALL

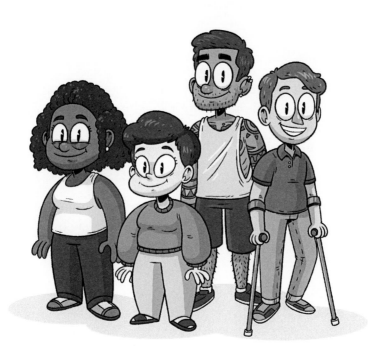

Let's talk about the word "normal."

For many, this word is the bane of their existence because it places upon all of us the pressure to conform to a societal expectation that is always shifting and changing. In the realm of eating, food, and nourishment, the word "normal" becomes a weapon used to sell products that can end up demeaning people, fueling comparison culture, and result in the creation of destructive food rules.

What is truly normal when it comes to nourishing our bodies and taking care of ourselves is simply doing what comes to us naturally. We are all born with the innate ability to recognize when we are hungry, what type and how much nourishment we need, and when we have had enough. Our genetics or the food environment in which we were raised can contribute to the differences seen in normal eating among different people.

The true normal relies on our ability to listen to the messages and cues of our incredible bodies as they let us know what we need to feel balanced and function optimally.

Compared to the *diet culture* definition of normal, this may seem revolutionary. After all, diet culture tells us to ignore the cues of our body, to cut out certain food groups, to tell ourselves "no" when we are craving something, and to restrict and limit our intake. The normal of diet culture is not concerned with taking care of your body so it can function well; it is only concerned with doing what it takes to achieve the societal image of health, physical fitness, and beauty.

According to Ellyn Satter, MS, RDN, MSSW:

> Normal eating is going to the table hungry and eating until you are satisfied. It is being able to choose food you enjoy and eat it and truly get enough of it—not just stop eating because you think you should.

> Normal eating is being able to give some thought to your food selection so you get nutritious food, but not being so wary and restrictive that you miss out on enjoyable food. Normal eating is giving yourself permission to eat sometimes because you are happy, sad, or bored, or just because it feels good.

> Normal eating is mostly three meals a day, or four or five, or it can be choosing to munch along the way. It is leaving some cookies on the plate because you know you can have some again tomorrow, or it is eating more now because they taste so wonderful.

> Normal eating is overeating at times, feeling stuffed

and uncomfortable. And it can be undereating at times and wishing you had more.

Normal eating is trusting your body to make up for your mistakes in eating.

Normal eating takes up some of your time and attention, but keeps its place as only one important area of your life. In short, normal eating is flexible. It varies in response to your hunger, your schedule, your proximity to food, and your feelings.[1, 2]

Ellyn Satter suggests that normal eating looks like:

- Normal eating is not having any food rules. It's being able to eat freely without considering your body shape, size, or appearance. It is having no feelings of guilt, shame, or remorse about the food choices you have made.
- Normal eating is being able to try a new food, or eat outside of the "recommended serving size" because your body tells you it needs more.
- Normal eating is being able to eat because you simply enjoy a certain food.
- Normal eating is knowing that no one food can negatively or positively change your body. You can stop being at war with your body and food.
- Normal is natural, normal is flexible, normal is balanced.
- Normal should set you free, not cage you in.

The Varying Degrees of Normal

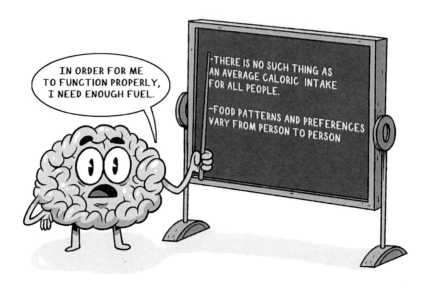

Diet culture limits the concept of normal, making it seem like an unobtainable goal for most individuals. The truth is, what is considered normal health, nutrition, and eating should be unbound, because it is different for every person and can change from day to day.

We are all born with having varying hunger and fullness levels. We have bodies that look different and function optimally in their own unique ways. Life experiences can cause alterations in all of these aspects. The amount and variety of food that people eat is greatly influenced by multiple factors, and there isn't one neat heading that we all fall under.

As another example, society gives the incorrect impression that there is an average required daily caloric intake, putting people in the mindset that they are either over- or undereating. An individual whose movement is made up of activities around the house will have different nourishment requirements than an avid athlete. Neither is overeating nor undereating. Each is nourishing themselves with the amount of food their body is communicating it needs for their particular lifestyle. Similarly, normal food patterns, rituals, and preferences vary from person to person. Someone who is recovered from an eating disorder and has healed their relationship with food does not have any food rules, and food is viewed as just food. There are no consequences or need for punishment for having a certain food. An individual is able to eat what feels good in the moment, and move on with their day. Chronic dieting is not normal, since nearly one in four dieters will progress to develop an eating disorder.[3]

Our culture attempts to categorize food as good or bad. It is true that some individuals may need to modify their food selection because of a medical condition; however, excluding whole food groups for everyone across the board in an attempt to be healthy is unwarranted. What is considered normal eating for one might be unhealthy for another, and neither individual needs to make changes or compromises to match the other.

Misinterpreting Normal

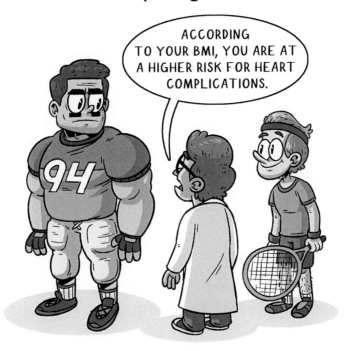

If normal is actually more natural, how did everything become so complicated?

A lot of the misinterpretation of normal comes from diet culture. In today's society, restricting, dieting, or having disordered eating behaviors is considered to be normal. The only thing normal about these things is that almost everyone engages in such behaviors at some point in their life.

However, normal and common are not the same thing. Something that is common can still be incredibly harmful and based on false information and pseudoscience. We are bombarded with media messages and advertising misinformation describing the "evils" of various foods and food groups. They promise that getting rid of these evils will lead to happiness, attractiveness, wealth, fulfillment, and love. Advertisers and companies rely on all of us wanting such things, and if we just cut out this, buy that, lose this, or change that, our desires will come to fruition. We jump on the dieting bandwagon with the intention of improving our lives, but because we were lied to, end up dissatisfied and disappointed. We then jump on board the next fad, hoping it will deliver the promises we did not receive before.

The dieting cycle continues and messes up the individual's relationship with food, nourishment, their body, happiness, and self-worth. People are taught to ignore their body's signals and hunger cues. Eating becomes stressful and complicated because now there are so many rules. Not surprisingly, all the rules change every few years. Something that was vilified becomes great, and something new becomes vilified. It makes eating extraordinarily confusing until people learn to go back to the way things were, before society jumbled everything up: listen to your body, listen to your cravings, listen to your hunger signals, and nourish yourself accordingly. When you take care of your body in a way that values your well-being and lifestyle, your body will be where it is naturally meant to be. When we legalize food and it becomes neutral, our reaction to it becomes neutral too.

Everyone is looking outside for simple answers to nutrition, when the answers have always been within.

The Role of Lab Tests in Defining Normal

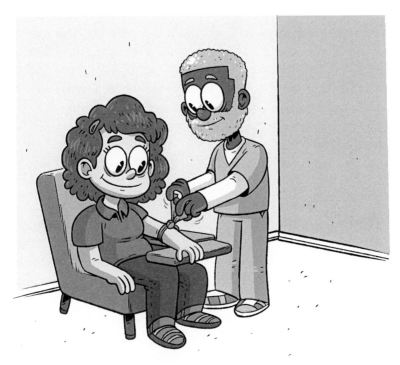

The concept of normal becomes even more complicated when clinicians, registered dietitians, and medical professionals consider patient lab test results in an attempt to assess their nutrition and health.

Lab tests can be valuable. They can provide a more accurate picture of what is going on in the individual's body, as opposed to making assumptions about their health based on their physical appearance, or the arbitrary measurement of BMI. Individuals with different body shapes and sizes may find that their labs do not reflect anything relevant about their nutritional status.

Our bodies are remarkable at working hard internally to compensate for any nutritional deficits. For example, an individual with anorexia nervosa who is at a weight too low for their body to function optimally can have normal lab tests. They may then utilize this information as evidence that they don't need to make any changes to their lifestyle or dietary intake. However, there could be a lot going on that is not reflected in their labs—forgetfulness, sleeping problems, dizziness, light-headedness, etc.

On the flip side, an individual who has a higher BMI may be told they need to lose weight or that they are unhealthy. All of their lab test results and physical exams, though, will be normal, showing they have no health issues. Is it possible to be healthy and have all your labs be normal and still be living in a larger body? Absolutely. Is it possible to be restricting and malnourished and have all your labs be normal? Again, absolutely.

Labs do not reveal weight cycling, weight stigma, restriction, or even a history of trauma.

There are nutritional parameters that only lab tests can reveal. If an individual is nourishing themselves appropriately, the expectation is that lab results will indicate that their body is in balance. In such an individual, blood cell counts, electrolytes, and hormone levels will likely be in the normal range. However, lab results do not indicate what the individual's relationship with food is like and whether they engage in any disordered eating behaviors. Lab results, then, should be used as one tool, and not as the definitive determinant of one's health status— just like you wouldn't only lay your eyes on somebody and determine whether they are nutritionally healthy.

Even the standard for what constitutes a normal lab result is subjective. Not everyone responds the same to deviations in blood test results. For example, the normal range for creatinine is 0.75–1.2 mg/dL. For a muscular young man, a level of 1.2 might be normal, but for someone with low muscle mass, a 1.2 creatinine might be read as "normal," but actually reflects 50 percent renal function loss.

Laboratory tests can be part of your clinical assessment of a patient. Clinicians typically look at blood cell counts, comprehensive metabolic panels, thyroid function tests, endocrine function, liver function tests, lipid panels, hormone levels, and vitamin D levels.

A CBC, or Complete Blood Cell Count, measures an individual's red and white blood cell count. This can help show you if the bone marrow is producing enough cells. Other lab tests show electrolyte levels. Two electrolytes specifically looked at are sodium and potassium levels. Individuals who abuse laxatives or diuretics, or who self-induce vomiting, may have low levels of these electrolytes. Amylase can also be elevated in those with self-induced vomiting (but this may not always be the most accurate test).

Low blood-glucose levels may indicate restrictive eating behaviors, as would decreased levels of the hormones testosterone and estrogen.

Labs are wonderful tools; however, they do not give us the entire picture. In order to find out how an individual relates to their body, to their hunger and fullness cues, how they nourish themselves, their self-worth, self-image, and exercise habits, it is important to ask many questions about their personal history as well as their family history.

Do You Look "Normal"?

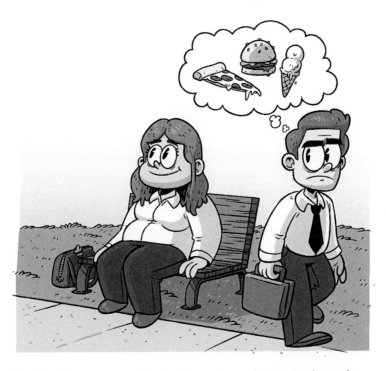

Think of your own ideals honestly and genuinely. Ask yourself what it is you believe you can assume about a person based on their appearance. It is an all-too-common practice for humans to make quick judgments about one another, believing that they can decipher an individual's health, intelligence, worth, personality, past, present, and future based on how they appear physically. The harmful impact of this has resulted in issues with racism, sexism, and discrimination against numerous minority populations throughout history. To be discriminated against because of appearance is nothing new.

Weight bias is a negative and weight-related attitude, belief, assumption, or judgment toward individuals who are overweight or ob*se.[4] This bias is demonstrated routinely on social media, in movies, television, and advertisements.

Our diet and appearance-obsessed culture makes it clear what bodies are valued and what bodies are not. They associate positive attributes to people living in smaller bodies or "fit" bodies, and attribute negative qualities to those in larger bodies. Without even thinking about it, people may automatically assume an individual in a larger body is lazy.

These assumptions have harmful results. Weight discrimination has increased 66 percent in the last decade, and occurs more frequently than gender or age discrimination.[5] Youth who are bullied by their peers for living in larger bodies are two to three times more likely to experience suicidal thoughts and behaviors than those who are not victimized.[6]

The beliefs about what is normal, and the societal pressures of conforming to specific BMI measurements, lab test results, appearances, or size, are dangerous and hurtful. These beliefs are so embedded in our culture that they often go unnoticed. Individuals who have a body size or shape that doesn't fit a cookie-cutter image are the ones being harmed.

A Normal Diagnosis:
How Appearance Bias Impacts Treatment

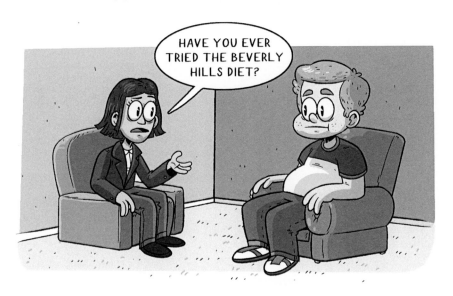

Let's be candid. Any clinician or medical professional who has weight bias is dangerous, especially to those struggling with disordered eating.

A 2014 study published in the *International Journal of Eating Disorders* found that 35 percent of clinicians reported feeling uncomfortable caring for larger bodies, 56 percent observed negative comments while caring for larger bodies, 29 percent reported colleagues having negative attitudes toward individuals living in larger bodies, and 42 percent believe that even certain clinicians have negative stereotypes pertaining to individuals living in higher-weight bodies.[7]

These numbers can be seen not only in professionals' attitudes toward patients living in larger bodies, but also in the arrangement of the medical offices themselves. Examples are furniture that is not comfortable for individuals living in larger bodies, or a scale that only goes up to a certain number.

These professionals may not be trained in eating disorders, or nutrition in general, and possibly have unresolved issues with food and their own body which they project onto patients.

One outcome of this lack of training is an overreliance on the measurement of BMI as an indicator of health. As a culture, we are obsessed with BMI as well as with the idea that weight equals health, and therefore normal BMI equals health too. As mentioned in chapter 4, this completely ignores individual factors such as genetics and body composition. Some people are meant to be tall, some people are meant to be short, some people are meant to have blue eyes, some green eyes, and some people are meant to be fat while others are meant to be skinny. This is just a representation of our unique genetic makeup, which we have no control over. However, when BMI is the main instrument being used to measure health, much can go wrong.

There have been situations in which individuals living in larger bodies with atypical anorexia nervosa have been told by doctor after doctor to cut down on calories, assuming that because they are in a larger body, they are overeating. In reality, these individuals may display all of the symptoms of anorexia nervosa once their food intake and nutritional balance are assessed. When a trained clinician or medical professional finally sees the whole picture, and advises the patient to eat more and eat more consistently, the patient is understandably shocked and confused. Every other doctor had simply looked at their BMI and told them to eat less without looking at the fact that they were eating so little it was hurting their overall health.

Weight bias in the medical community is so off-putting that some individuals in larger bodies, who truly have a health issue, will not seek medical care. They do not want to be judged and stigmatized for their body size, shape, and appearance. There have been many instances of individuals not feeling comfortable going to their doctor when medical attention was needed, because they knew their weight would be blamed for any unrelated ailment. This experience can be traumatizing.

Weight bias is not well understood amongst healthcare providers. They are often unaware that weight stigma is traumatic, and the stress an individual experiences as a result can cause disease, distress, and dysfunction.

Consider the higher-weight patient who needs a knee replacement, but is denied this medically therapeutic procedure until they lose weight. The patient is told that exercise is part of a healthy lifestyle. If they are in pain when they walk, they are put in a complete no-win situation; they cannot have the surgery to take away that pain until they lose the weight.

It is important to point out these are not incompetent medical professionals, or individuals who are intentionally behaving maliciously. These are well-educated and informed individuals who are simply expressing the weight bias that has sadly become commonplace in our culture. This weight bias comes from the lack of understanding that a person can have health at any size.[8]

When a doctor, however competent, is weight-biased, it leaves incredible room for error. These errors could include misdiagnoses, poor care, or a complete disregard of needing more information from the patient. Patients feel they will not be taken seriously, and oftentimes do not share their weight concerns out of fear of judgment.

The entire concept of "normal," whether you look at it medically, socially, or psychologically, is dangerous and unnecessary. Normal is a word that always implies comparison. After all, normal means measuring up against an average. The new normal is letting go of the concept of normal, and breaking the chains it places on you and your clients for having to fit a specific ideal or image. The new normal is that there is no normal.

Chapter 5 Notes

1. Ellyn Satter, *Secrets of Feeding a Healthy Family* (Madison, WI: Kelcy Press, 1983), 16.

2. Ellyn Satter, "What Is Normal Eating?" Ellyn Satter Institute (2018), https://www.ellynsatterinstitute.org/wp-content/uploads/2017/11/What-is-normal-eating-Secure.pdf.

3. "Statistics & Research on Eating Disorders," National Eating Disorders Association, accessed December 20, 2019, www.nationaleatingdisorders.org/statistics-research-eating-disorders.

4. Angela Alberga et al., "Weight bias: a call to action," *Journal of Eating Disorders* 4 (2016): 34.

5. R. Puhl et al., "Weight bias among professionals treating eating disorders: attitudes about treatment and perceived patient outcomes," *International Journal of Eating Disorders* 47, no. 1 (January 2014): 65–75, doi: 10.1002/eat 22186.

6. Meg H. Zeller et al., "Adolescent suicidal behavior across the excess weight status spectrum," *Ob*sity* 21, no. 5 (May 2013): 1039–1045, doi: 10.1002/oby.20084.

7. R. Puhl et al., "Weight bias among professionals."

8. Linda Bacon, *Health at Every Size: The Surprising Truth about Your Weight* (Dallas TX: BenBella Books, 2008).

CHAPTER 6

THE NUTRITION INTERVIEW: THE ROLE OF THE DIETITIAN

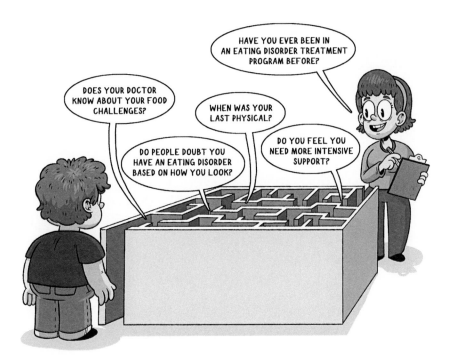

Armed with a better sense of awareness as to how to have important conversations with patients suffering from eating disorders, we can now focus on the nutrition interview. This interview helps doctors and other professionals diagnose and begin the process of treating patients, and assesses whether a referral to a specialized professional is warranted.

Think back to times in your own life when you kept something that was bothering you to yourself. As much as it ate away at you, the situation may have been so painful and close to your heart that you couldn't bring yourself to discuss it with anyone. The secretiveness made the situation grow in intensity, until someone may have asked, "Are you okay?" and this made the floodgates open.

This example illustrates why the nutrition interview is so important. People struggling with an eating disorder are often at a loss regarding how to talk about their situation. Asking the right questions can help facilitate this communication. Whether you are trained in eating disorders or not, asking specific questions (discussed below) can help shed light on the individual's burdensome secret.

Individuals struggling with eating disorders are often paralyzed by fear, and this can pull them in opposite directions. One voice may tell them they cannot continue to live this way and need help, while another voice may tell them to stay in control by staying in hiding. After all, their eating disorder is their companion that has helped them survive feelings of discomfort. Talking about it may allow someone to take their "life preserver" away.

The constant push and pull of these two voices or thought patterns builds up like a pressure cooker. Therefore, not proceeding gently when working with these individuals could lead to an explosive mess. Treading cautiously with questions about their eating, weight history, exercise, health, and any prior treatment slowly releases this pressure. Allowing the individual to take the lead in telling their story gives them a sense of control and builds trust, paving the path to receiving the help they desperately need.

Entering the Labyrinth

There are many directions a professional can take in this line of questioning. It is like walking through a maze with numerous paths, not knowing where you are going when you first begin, with each step taken determining the next step.

A nutrition interview begins with a standard line of questioning about the individual's physical health, dieting history, food rules, and thoughts about their body. One question naturally leads to the next. The only requirement is that these questions be asked with respect, curiosity, and kindness, not judgment.

This "maze" is also new for the individual struggling with an eating disorder. Having these conversations with you can be scary. Your line of questioning may feel threatening to them. What if they are an athlete on a scholarship, and they feel they need to maintain their extreme workout schedule to stay competitive? Might you take that, and their future dreams, away?

The Big Four

There is no shortage of possible questions to ask a person with an eating disorder. But generally, they can be broken down into the following four categories:

1. Past and Present Health
2. Past and Present Weight History and Eating Patterns
3. Past and Present Treatment
4. Personal Goals and Values

Each of these categories sheds light on the development of their eating disorder and their disordered behaviors. Information gathered here can lead to early and effective intervention, resulting in better outcomes.

Past and Present Health

An individual's physical assessment can teach you much more about their eating disorder than you may think. Most people consider an emaciated appearance to be the only physical indicator of an eating disorder. This can be one of many indicators, and it can often be unreliable. Individuals struggling with an eating disorder can present with diverse body shapes and sizes.

Consider the metaphor of our body as a car. What would happen if we deprived our car of the proper gasoline, lubrication, oil, or fluids? Not only would it not work properly, it would put stress on the entire machine, and it would try to compensate for the dysfunction. The same holds true for our bodies—when we don't fuel it properly for optimal performance, it puts stress on all our organs.

Engaging in disordered eating behaviors is like throwing a rock in a pond; it creates ripples that impact the individual physically, mentally, emotionally, socially, and spiritually. The type of eating disorder, and how long the individual has had the eating disorder for, can manifest a variety of symptoms and problems. These might include:

- Disturbed sleep (having difficulty falling asleep or staying asleep through the night)
- Thinning hair (noticing more hair loss on your pillow, on your brush, or in the shower; or a slowing of hair growth)
- Difficulty concentrating
- Trouble with maintaining a conversation
- Poor memory
- Mood changes
- Night sweats
- Menstrual irregularities and/or hormonal changes (having no period, or shorter periods with a lighter flow)

Asking the following questions can inform you about the individual's health status:

- When was your last physical?
- Have you had recent lab tests done? What were the results?
- Have you ever had a bone density test, or an EKG?
- Have you observed that your hair has thinned, that you are losing it easily, or that it has become dry or brittle?
- Have you noticed that your nails are breaking more easily?
- Does your skin continue to be dry despite using moisturizer?
- Do you have sleeping difficulties?
- Do you sweat during your sleep?
- Have you experienced any gastrointestinal issues, such as nausea, vomiting, constipation, bloating, abdominal pain, or diarrhea?
- Have you ever vomited blood?
- Do you bruise more easily?
- Do you feel cold all the time?
- Do you smoke cigarettes?
- Do you drink a lot of caffeine?
- Do you currently menstruate?
- At what age did you start menstruating?
- Typically, how many days is your cycle?

- Are your periods heavy, light, irregular?
- Has your menstrual cycle changed since engaging in these behaviors?
- Are you on hormone replacement therapy (HRT) or birth control pills?
- Have you experienced any change or difficulty in getting or maintaining an erection?

Some of these questions may be uncomfortable or inappropriate to ask; use your professional judgment regarding what is appropriate for your setting, profession, and position.

Past and Present Weight History and Eating Patterns

The answers to these questions can be the most indicative of concerning behaviors and beliefs. These questions are broken down into four subcategories.

Weight

Finding out an individual's weight history, and how they feel about it, can be very revealing. Some may casually mention weight increases or decreases throughout their life, while others can tell you exactly what their weight was at any given point in their life. It is important to notice not just what they say, but also how they say it. Are they apologetic about their weight? Are they afraid or anxious discussing their weight? Do they relate their worth to their weight? These observations provide a lot more insight than a simple number can.

You may ask the individual:

- What was your weight like growing up?
- Do you recall the weight range you were at when you began your disordered eating/diet?
- Do you weigh yourself?
- Do others comment on your weight?
- How often do you weigh yourself?
- How does the number on the scale make you feel?
- How does weighing yourself impact your day?

Body Image

Eating disorders are about much more than physical appearances, but that does not mean body image and self-image do not play a role. Important insight is gained by finding out how individuals view themselves and their body, and how this relates to their feelings of self-worth.

Some questions to ask are:

- How do you feel about your body?
- Do you often compare your appearance to others?
- Do you avoid looking at your body, or in the mirror? Do you dim the lights before you look at yourself?
- Do you try to hide your body with baggy clothes?
- Do you engage in frequent "body checking"?
- Do/have your family members/friends/coaches/doctors comment/commented on your body?
- What comments do your family members make about their own body/the bodies of others?

Physical Activity

Eating disorders can involve restrictive or compulsive eating behaviors, as well as exercising in an attempt to compensate for "extra" calories consumed, or to change physical appearance or weight. Obtaining information about exercise patterns can help you distinguish between an active individual or one who uses exercise in a disordered way.

You can inquire:

- Do you currently engage in physical activity? If so, how often and for how long?
- Do you feel you have to exercise?
- Do you feel compelled to exercise if you eat certain foods, or a certain amount of food?
- Do you engage in physical activity for the enjoyment of moving your body, or is it a way for you to control your weight and shape?
- Are you able to take days off from exercise if you are tired or sick?

- Do you avoid exercise/movement because of how you feel about your body?
- Do you avoid movement because loved ones and/or healthcare providers have asked you to incorporate it into your regimen?

Nutrition and Food Rules

Learning an individual's beliefs about food and nutrition and how they nourish themselves is a quick way to determine whether they have a healthy relationship with food and their body.

Some questions you may ask:

- When was your first diet?
- What was the reason you started dieting?
- Was there a person who influenced you to begin dieting?
- Do you follow diet trends now?
- What are your food rules?
- Do you have a list of safe and unsafe foods?
- Are there any food rituals you engage in?
- How long does it take for you to eat your meals/snacks?
- Are you vegetarian or vegan?
- Do you only eat at certain times of the day?
- Do you deprive yourself of certain foods?
- Do you use food to punish or reward yourself?
- Do you eat and purge?
- Do you eat and spit?
- Do you take laxatives and/or diuretics?
- Do you eat more when you are stressed or upset?
- Do you eat out of boredom?
- Do you consume caffeinated beverages or water to alter your appetite?
- Does preparing food make you anxious?
- Do you like to cook but never try what you make?
- What proteins/carbohydrates/fats do you eat? How much? How often?

Past and Present Treatment History

Asking questions about an individual's treatment experience includes any eating disorder treatment, as well as basic medical checkups. You may encounter individuals who have not only had no previous treatment for their disorder, they are not at a point to even acknowledge they have a disorder! Learning about their previous experiences with doctors, tests they may have done, and/or any other treatments is a great place to start the conversation.

If they have had previous treatment by a professional in the same field as you, they are likely coming to you because they feel they did not receive the care they needed elsewhere. Knowing the details of what worked and didn't work with the previous clinician will enable you to become more attuned with the treatment you provide.

The point of these following questions is not to focus on the shortcomings of previous clinicians, but rather to fine-tune your interventions to the needs of your client.

Here are some sample questions to ask:

- Does your doctor know about your food challenges?
- How does your doctor respond to any such challenges?
- Has your doctor ever made any dietary suggestions based on your body weight?
- Have you ever been diagnosed with an eating disorder?
- Have you ever been in an eating disorder–treatment program?
- Have you ever been hospitalized for any other reason?
- Do you feel clinicians you have worked with in the past were helpful?
- What was helpful, and what are some areas for improvement?

Personal Goals and Values

Exploring an individual's goals and values can help provide them with a broader life perspective. It can offer them hope and help them see what the future can hold when they are healed. It also helps create rapport, making them be more open to your nutrition interview.

Some questions you can ask:

- What do you most value in life?
- What do you most value in yourself?
- What would you most value in a friend?
- Is the way you are living your life now aligned with those values?
- What do you want to be when you grow up?
- Where would you like to be in one year? In five years?
- What would you like to be doing?
- Will the way you are living your life now lead you to that desired future?

When individuals feel cared for and not judged, they are more likely to open up to you about their experiences with food and their bodies. Therefore, the most important rule to remember when executing the nutrition interview is to do so in a supportive and nonjudgmental way. Coming from a place of curiosity will have you walking on the path of exploration with your client. Together you can gain insight and work toward meaningful resolutions. The nutrition interview will guide both of you through the maze, and ultimately lead to helpful and appropriate interventions, treatment, and/or appropriate referral sources.

CHAPTER 7

SCORCHED EARTH: EATING DISORDERS' IMPACT ON THE BODY

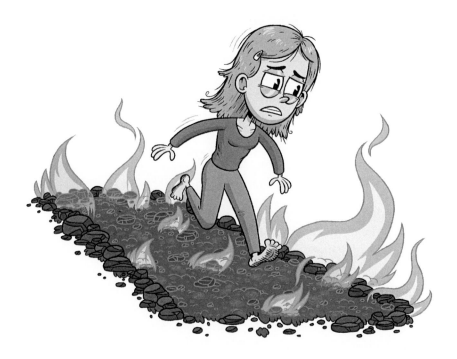

In the previous chapter, we discussed the different types of eating disorders and some of the symptoms common to each. Because eating disorders can present in many different forms, they are not only hard to diagnose, but equally difficult to treat. However, each one is a parasitic monster, aggressively attacking many organs simultaneously. Although everyone will have different physiologic changes related to malnutrition, one cannot optimally coexist with a parasite.

Eating disorders sound relatively benign—after all, they are just about eating. But since eating is pivotal for survival, one's eating poorly can have serious consequences. Eating disorders usually start out subtly and with what appear to be good intentions, such as being "healthy." As a result, they almost always catch people off guard. Sufferers and their family members frequently comment that they did not see the changes for a long time, and when they did, it had already become a serious situation. On the other hand, with extreme dieting and exercise, eating disorders can be fulminant at the outset. Regardless of how they start, the resulting malnutrition is a global assault on the body. These terrible illnesses affect all body systems, sparing none in their ruthless pursuit.

Let's start by clarifying what malnutrition is. It is not only the avoidance of food, but the avoidance of enough food, including fluids. How much food and fluid an individual needs is dependent on their activities of daily living, movement, and a host of other variables. Our bodies are not math equations; they have many complex mechanisms and feedback systems that determine metabolism, size, shape, muscle mass, fat mass, and weight.

My colleague Marci Evans, MS, RDN, CEDRD-S, explains below how the expression "calories in vs. calories out" is meaningless:

> These kinds of dieting messages are useless because it assumes you eat the same exact number of calories every day and that subtracting a specific number of calories will lead to a consistent caloric deficit. That's not how it works when you are human. This message is also harmful because it is misleading. It gives the false notion that if you count your calories precisely (spoiler: you cannot) and exercise enough willpower (spoiler: willpower dooms us all), you can simply write up a math calculation to get yourself to your chosen weight. None of this is possible and here is why: Of course our body weight is impacted by what we eat and how our body uses that fuel. But it is also influenced by a host of other complex mechanisms that we have very little control over, thanks to the genetics passed along from our parents. Most importantly, attempts to decrease intake and increase output creates a massive change in our physiology that undermines efforts to down-regulate our weight. This includes but is not limited to:

1. **Basal Metabolic Rate**—This accounts for about 70 percent of our metabolic activity and decreases as weight is lost.

2. **Appetite Hormones like Leptin and Ghrelin**—Turns out that, as a person loses weight, the body shifts the production of these hormones to encourage increased intake.

3. **Changes in the Reward System in the Brain**—For the neuroscience geeks, it is particularly related to the orbital frontal cortex, which is related to the reward pathways in our brain making sure we seek out more food and don't die of famine.

Consequently, when we try to alter calories in and calories out, there are a host of other "numerics" that step in to complicate the equation. However, an important fact is that the way and the degree to which these responses happen in your body is outside of your control and largely dictated by genetics.

People often forget their genetics, or want to change their genetics, which they are not able to do. Our genes are our genes, just like our eye color is the eye color we were born with. When we put our body through unnatural and extreme measures, we become more fixated on our food intake and movement, which can lead to bigger problems (i.e. disordered eating/eating disorders).

Eating disorders ravage all body functions—from organs to bones to the brain to the heart to fat tissue—everything.

All tissues in the body need food and fluids. Water, electrolytes, micronutrients, proteins, calories, carbohydrates, fat, vitamins, minerals, and more support structures and chemical reactions to make the brain, muscles, and body work optimally.

When any of these is in short supply, the body does its best to adjust and adapt. However, it can only do so if the degree of deficit is not too great. If the loss becomes too extreme or too prolonged, the body will reach a point where it can no longer counteract the deficit and meet the demands of the body.

Let's discuss how eating disorders impact various organs.

Healing the Broken Heart

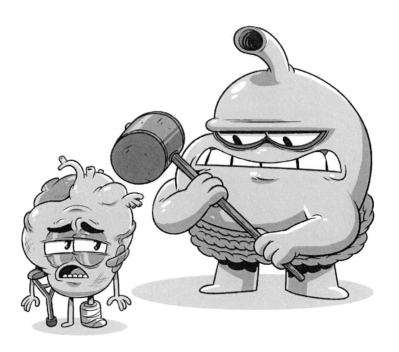

We all know that the heart is the life source of our body. It is a muscle that works 24/7, every second of a person's life. Just as with any machine, its parts wear down with time and use. However, this wear and tear is significantly expedited when illness or malnutrition comes into play.

Bradycardia (slowing down of the heart rate) is one of the first adjustments the heart will make when faced with malnutrition. To get a picture of how much energy it takes for the heart to beat, imagine yourself squeezing a ball strongly and rapidly every second of every day for an undetermined amount of days. That's a lot of energy!

The brain is aware of this, and in times of deficit, will send a signal via the vagus nerve (one of the cranial nerves that influences the heart, lungs, and digestive system) to slow down these organs. The heart can slow down from a normal range of sixty to a hundred beats per minute to as low as twenty beats per minute. As a point of reference, a well-trained "healthy" athlete's heart can beat as low as fifty beats per minute. However, this slow a heart rate isn't always a sign of fitness and may indicate there is more to the story.[1] The result of a slowed heart rate is that not enough oxygen reaches organs, leading to some of the following symptoms: fainting, dizziness, fatigue, chest pain, confusion, and exhaustion.

Malnutrition can also result in the muscle of the heart shrinking, and its inside chamber size to decrease. When the heart beats slower, less blood is pumped per beat, so it has to work harder to get the same work done. Hence, the heart becomes strained stuck between needing to simultaneously slow down and speed up.

If that were not enough to weaken the heart, malnutrition from eating disorders affects the electrical activity of the heart. The electrical activity of the heart conducts its muscle contraction. This dysregulation results in dysrhythmias (abnormal heartbeat) that can become severe enough to cause death. An ECG/EKG can detect this and should be part of the cardiac workup of a person with malnutrition. These rhythm changes can make one feel like their heart is racing and beating stronger (called palpitations), or can occur without symptoms, be sudden, and be fatal.

The heart pumps blood throughout the body, hence a weak and strained heart impacts blood pressure. As the body is trying to save energy, blood is pumped primarily to vital organs. As a result, people will often report that their extremities (fingers, toes, hands, and feet) are cold. Eventually, the whole body becomes cold.

This can be demonstrated by a capillary refill delay. You can test this by squeezing your hand into a fist for a few seconds, opening it, and seeing how fast pink color returns to the hand. If it takes more than two seconds or so, it can be an indication of this delay.

It is a good idea to make patients aware of their altered bodily functions. For example, let the patient do the capillary refill time with you. Allow them to see how fast your (the clinician's) blood returns, and how theirs is delayed. Or let the client feel the change in their pulse from lying down to standing.

If adequate blood is not reaching body tissues, it results in a bluish-purple hue to the skin called acrocyanosis. This hue can indicate that the body is having difficulty pumping blood from the heart to that area of the body. Checking blood pressure and pulse when lying down, and comparing it to blood pressure and pulse when sitting, is another way to check for the adequacy of blood volume. If the values are significantly different, it can be an indicator of cardiac dysfunction, as a result of malnutrition and/or dehydration.

Common cardiac symptoms seen in people with eating disorders:

- Heart suddenly beating fast/heart palpitations*
- Slow heartbeat in a nonathlete (under sixty beats/min)*
- Low blood pressure in a nonathlete (systolic under ninety, diastolic under fifty)*
- V-tach (ventricular tachycardia)*
- Inverted T-waves (abnormal ECG/EKG)*
- Irregular Q-T interval
- Feeling the heart "skips beats" or "jump"*
- Chest pain*
- Shortness of breath or trouble breathing*
- Trouble exercising*
- Swelling in the hands and feet*
- Cold extremities*
- Delayed capillary refill*

Physician notification and involvement strongly advised.

Brain Drain

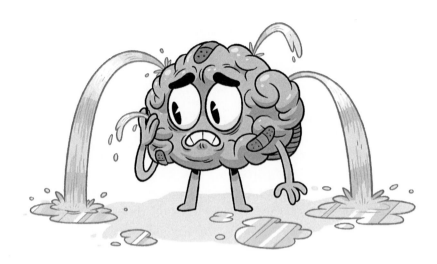

The heart takes its instructions from the brain. The brain is the organ that exerts centralized control over all organs in the body. Just as with the heart, the brain does not function well when malnourished.

When first malnourished, the brain goes through structural changes. It can lead to the loss of myelin, a fatty covering of brain nerves, decreasing the speed of messages sent between nerves. This loss can occur early with the restriction of food. In contrast, the devastating disease multiple sclerosis also involves the loss of myelin in the brain and central nervous system, but due to causes not related to malnutrition.

As malnutrition is prolonged, more brain nerves die. These brain nerves, or neurons, run the brain's "communication highway." A process called pruning is expedited in malnutrition. Pruning refers to the brain's self-cleaning process of removing damaged neurons. In malnutrition, pruning begins to occur more quickly as neurons die off faster. MRIs of individuals with severe anorexia nervosa sometimes show the individual's brain looking more like that of an individual with Alzheimer's disease.

In addition to neuron loss, there is also a depletion of neurotransmitters (chemical messengers of the brain). Neurotransmitters help regulate mood, anxiety, and compulsive behaviors. Most common is the depletion of the neurotransmitter serotonin. Serotonin is involved in mood and anxiety regulation. If an already stressed brain is then depleted of mood-supporting neurotransmitters, the individual's recovery process becomes more complicated. If there is a genetic predisposition for mood and anxiety disorders, malnutrition can intensify this. Recovery may require additional psychiatric support.

Aside from mood, the actual neurological functioning of the brain is altered by an eating disorder. Several studies using functional MRIs have documented that brains of those with anorexia nervosa have different brain activity compared to those without.[2] This altered brain function is proven to lead to worsened eating disorder behaviors, because the eating disorder has changed how the individual's mind functions and processes information. These alterations become more entrenched as the disorder continues to be untreated.

As discussed before, cardiac complications decrease blood flow to the brain. When the brain does not get enough blood, oxygen, and glucose, it can lead to feelings of light-headedness and passing out (syncope).

An impaired brain leads to an impaired mind. Common symptoms related to the brain seen in people with eating disorders are:

- Difficulty concentrating*
- Poor memory*
- Falling asleep or extreme fatigue during the daytime (e.g. at school or work)*
- Trouble falling or staying asleep at night*
- Increase in depression or anxiety*
- Hurting oneself by cutting, scratching, burning, or other forms of self-inflicted injury*

Physician notification and involvement strongly advised.

Sweet Nothings

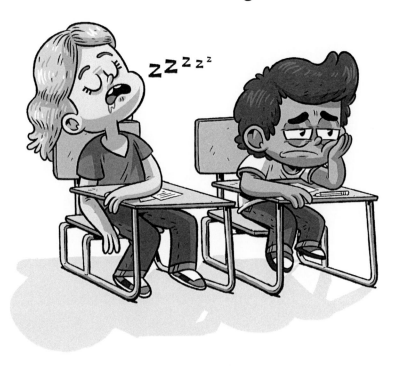

It is important to note that the body's response to refeeding the malnourished client is reaching a hypermetabolic state. This is when the metabolism, or rate of caloric expenditure, becomes faster by eating.[3] The solution to combating this accelerated metabolism is to eat even more food, which is often easier said than done.

Malnutrition also results in the depletion of the brain's primary energy source, glucose. This can lead to low blood sugar, or hypoglycemia. If the body detects a drop in glucose, it will convert glycogen stored in the liver into glucose to refeed the brain; however, if not repleted, these stores eventually run out as well. Glucose is the preferred fuel for the brain. In periods of severe deficit, the brain can adapt to using ketones for fuel. Ketones are formed from the breakdown of fat. A tell-tale sign of the body being in ketosis (using ketones because of a deficit of glucose) is having foul breath.

Despite the demonization of sugar by society, all carbohydrates break down into glucose, and it remains a fact that the brain thrives on glucose. In fact, severe hypoglycemia can result in seizures and coma, and increases the risk for sudden death.

Common symptoms related to hypoglycemia seen in people with eating disorders are:

- Difficulty concentrating*
- Poor memory*
- Feeling tired/having low energy*
- Feeling inappropriately cold or hot*

Physician notification and involvement strongly advised.

On the flip side, in clients with binge-eating disorder or bulimia nervosa, it is not uncommon to have insulin resistance. It is good practice to test for hemoglobin A1c, even in clients who have a normal blood glucose level.

Floods and Droughts

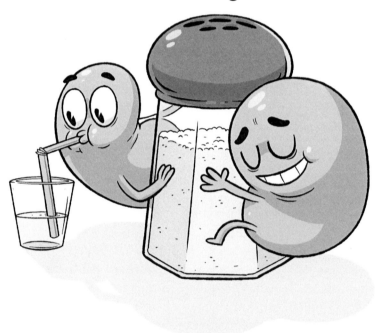

Dehydration can cause major havoc on the body's systems. A major responsibility of the kidneys is to regulate hydration status. When someone is dehydrated, the kidneys will hold on to more sodium. Sodium attracts water, allowing the kidneys to hold on to more water and rehydrate the body.

In order to compensate for holding on to more sodium, the kidneys excrete potassium. If potassium is already being lost as a result of client's using laxatives, diuretics, or purging, the dehydrated body will hold on to even more sodium.[4] The consequence of chronic dehydration from purging can be a condition called pseudo-Bartter syndrome, also known as secondary hyperaldosteronism. This is when the affinity for sodium causes the body to hold on to as much water as possible. The resulting edema (body's retaining of water) can cause the client to gain ten or more pounds over a course of a few days. Pseudo-Bartter syndrome can also cause water to leak into the abdomen (called ascites), or into the lungs, causing pulmonary edema. Treatment for this needs to be done in the hospital, because complications of low potassium can be cardiac arrhythmia, pulmonary edema, and cardiac arrest (heart attack).

In addition to blood pressure, skin turgor or skin elasticity can be checked to assess for dehydration: Grasp the skin on the back of the hand with two fingers so that it is tented up. Release the skin in a few seconds, and allow it to return to normal. A delay in the skin returning to normal is a sign of dehydration. Lack of skin turgor can be seen with mild dehydration.

Individuals with eating disorders tend to drink a lot of water to suppress their appetite. They may also "water-load" before weigh-ins to fake clinicians into believing any weight gain is due to better food intake versus the water they just drank. The excess intake of water and water-loading can dilute the body's electrolytes and lead to hyponatremia (low body sodium). If sodium levels get too low, serious consequences can occur such as fatigue, nausea, vomiting, headache, confusion, muscle cramps, seizures, or a coma. Repleting sodium too quickly can also have morbidity and mortality risks including death, if not closely monitored.

Common symptoms of dehydration seen in people with eating disorders are:

- Dizziness or feeling like one is going to pass out*

- Dry mouth*
- Headache/confusion*
- Muscle cramps*
- Fatigue*
- Nausea and vomiting*
- Dry skin*
- Poor skin turgor*

*Physician notification and involvement strongly advised.

That Gut Feeling

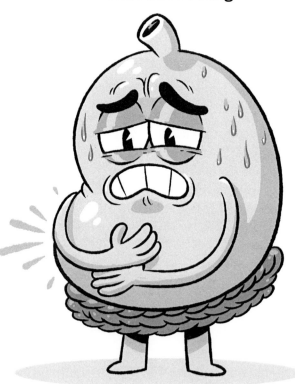

The gastrointestinal tract is affected by eating disorders in numerous ways. Frequent purging can cause tearing of the lining of the stomach and esophagus, leading to a GI bleed. A minor tear may show up as bright-red blood when vomiting, or the blood can travel down the intestines, leading to dark or black stools. A large tear or rupture of the esophagus can also occur, which can be life-threatening.

Frequent vomiting can also lead to gastroesophageal reflux disease (GERD). Prolonged self-induced vomiting loosens the sphincter muscle where the stomach and esophagus meet. This makes it easier for the acid from the stomach to travel up to the esophagus and cause irritation and burning of the esophageal lining. Over time, the exposure of acid to the esophagus can lead to changes in the lining of the esophagus, leading to a pre-cancerous condition called Barrett's esophagus. If not addressed, this can later turn into esophageal cancer.[5]

It is not uncommon for people with bulimia nervosa to be able to vomit spontaneously and effortlessly.

People who engage in binge-eating behavior can also damage their gastrointestinal tract. Large volumes of food consumed can stretch the stomach to the point that the supply of blood vessels to the stomach are cut off. This can cause stomach tissue to die. The distention caused by the large amount of food consumed can also make the stomach rupture, a life-threatening occurrence.

Another condition, gastroparesis, can occur as a result of insufficient food intake. Gastroparesis refers to the slowing down of the emptying of the stomach. This happens as a consequence of vagal activation from malnutrition as the body strives to spare calories. This can be especially problematic as individuals begin to eat enough food again. It takes a while for gastroparesis to resolve, leading to feelings of uncomfortable fullness. Clinicians need to be aware of this complication and support the client through this stage, which will eventually resolve with continued feeding. Providing nutrition in liquid form may help ease the symptoms of gastroparesis.

The prolonged use of laxatives can cause havoc in the large intestine. This can lead to the colon becoming used to the laxatives, making bowel movements almost impossible without them.

Oral health is also impacted by eating disorders. Inadequate fluid intake can lead to dry mouth, and the mouth needs plenty of saliva to prevent tooth decay. The likelihood of cavities is increased with binge-eating behavior due to the type of foods usually binged on. With vomiting, the acid from the stomach will eventually eat away at the enamel of the teeth, increasing tooth sensitivity and the risk for cavity formation.

The gut microbiome plays an important role in the health of the GI tract. The microbiome refers to the bacteria, microbes, and viruses that normally live in our GI tract. Interestingly, there are more bacterial cells in our body than there are human cells. Everyone has a unique gut microbiome. The gut bacteria produce enzymes that support digestion. The microbiome also affects the immune system, cognition, mood, and an individual's metabolic rate. A lack of caloric intake and food variety diminishes the production of beneficial bacteria in the microbiome. Clients with eating disorders typically complain of stomachaches, bloating, cramping, and constipation. This is related to malnutrition, and the impact of malnutrition on the gut microbiome. Consuming a varied diet ensures our gut microbiome will continue to flourish. This will support optimal digestion and bowel movement regularity.

Common symptoms of gastrointestinal distress seen in people with eating disorders are:

- Constipation or difficulty having a bowel movement*
- Stomachache or abdominal pain*
- Blood in the vomit or in the stools*
- Throwing up something that looks like coffee grounds*
- Chronic gas and bloating*
- Chronic belching *
- Chronic nausea*
- GERD (gastroesophageal reflux disease)*

Physician notification and involvement strongly advised.

Gotta Love Your Liver

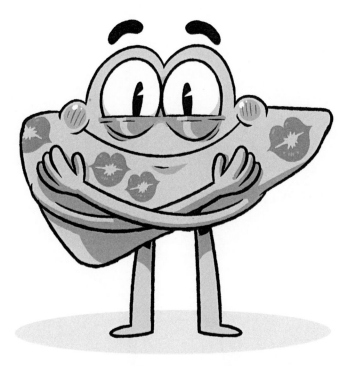

Hepatitis refers to the inflammation of the liver. Restricting calories or malnutrition can result in starvation hepatitis. In malnutrition, the liver will break down to provide the body with needed protein and calories. This can lead to elevated liver enzymes (AST and ALT) seen on a blood test. Clients are often surprised to realize these elevated liver enzymes can mean they are "eating their own liver" to compensate for their lack of food intake.

Refeeding hepatitis occurs when the liver becomes inflamed as a result of being refed too quickly. Dietitians/clinicians can prevent this by appropriately calculating the client's caloric needs and the percentage of calories to be provided in the form of carbohydrates.

A clinician can distinguish between starvation and refeeding hepatitis based on when they occur. Refeeding hepatitis usually takes a while to develop during the repair of nutrition deficit. Both starvation and refeeding hepatitis can be managed with proper treatment and do not generally result in lasting or permanent liver damage.

A Bloody Mess

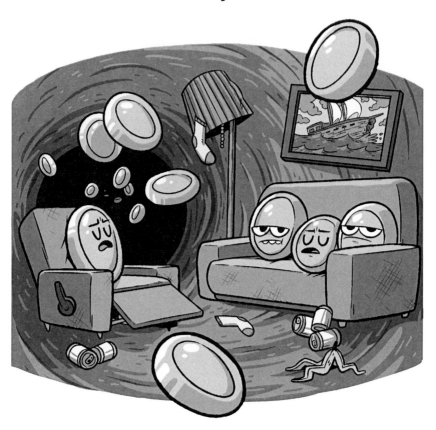

Malnutrition also affects the formation of the blood cells, including white blood cells, red blood cells, and platelets.

Prolonged malnutrition will lead to bone marrow suppression, decreasing the production of blood cells. The body is normally able to replenish any blood lost. However, patients with eating disorders who may experience blood loss will not be able to replenish their stores because of the suppression of their bone marrow, increasing the chances of their needing a blood transfusion.

The depletion of white blood cells can lead to an increased risk of infection. Because of the impaired immune system seen in starved patients, such patients with an infection may not develop a fever response.

The depletion of red blood cells can lead to anemia and its

accompanying symptoms. Low iron intake can also contribute to low red blood–cell levels.

The depletion of platelets can decrease clotting function, and lead to life-threatening severe bleeding. Low platelet levels make it easier for patients to bruise.

Common symptoms of low blood counts seen in people with eating disorders are:

- Easy bruising*
- Feeling tired or fatigued*
- Lack of energy*

Physician notification and involvement strongly advised.

Hot or Cold

The body maintains temperature within a relatively narrow range. We all know that even a two-degree fever can feel quite uncomfortable. As discussed in the heart section, a loss of body temperature is often the result of the body working to save energy, and pumping blood primarily to vital organs. As a result, people will often report that their extremities (fingers, toes, hands, and feet) are cold. A body temperature of ninety-six degrees or below is called hypothermia. Those with hypothermia feel constantly and achingly cold. Severely low body temperature poses a risk for death.

In an attempt to preserve body heat, lanugo can grow on the face and body. Lanugo is fine, soft hair seen on fetuses. This marker of malnutrition goes away with nutrition restoration.

Common symptoms of temperature fluctuations seen in people with eating disorders are:

- Feeling cold often*
- Blue fingers or toes*
- Facial or bodily lanugo*
- "Hot flashes" or sweating not related to exercise*

Physician notification and involvement strongly advised.

Boobs, Bones, and Breaks

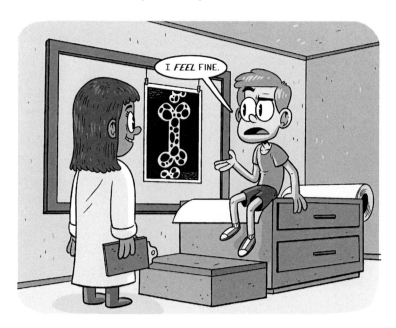

Malnutrition also alters sex hormones. The more severe the malnutrition, the more intense the decline of these hormones. This happens as a means for species preservation. When the brain detects that the body's energy reserve is inadequate to maintain a pregnancy, these changes occur. The brain decreases estrogen (estradiol) production in estrogen-based bodies (cis females, some trans males, nonbinary individuals), and decreases testosterone production in testosterone-based bodies (cis males, some trans females and nonbinary individuals). Decreased sex hormones cause a decrease in sex drive. In addition, in estrogen-based bodies, and/or in people who menstruate, the decrease in estradiol affects the lining of the uterus to an extent that pregnancy may or may not be possible.[6, 7, 8]

The two most obvious signs of lowered sex hormones in people with a uterus are a decrease in breast size, and the loss of the menstrual cycle (called secondary amenorrhea). In younger estrogen-based bodies who have not yet had a period, the menstrual cycle may be delayed indefinitely (called primary amenorrhea). In testosterone-based bodies, the classic symptom of diminished sex hormones is the loss of sex drive and erectile dysfunction.

A loss of sex drive was a common complaint in the first study ever done on starvation. At the close of World War II, a group of cis men in the army volunteered to do this study that lasted six months. A common complaint among participants was the loss of not only sex drive, but almost any interest or attraction to potential sexual partners.[9]

It is important to point out that malnutrition is not always 100 percent effective in preventing pregnancy, even with amenorrhea. Eating disorders are not a good form of birth control, and malnourished individuals can get pregnant.

Serum estradiol and testosterone levels should be checked in people with eating disorders, even in individuals who may be on prescription hormone medications.

Another consequence of low sex hormone levels in all genders is a loss of bone density. Normal sex hormone levels are required to maintain bone density. Most of skeletal bone development occurs during adolescence, ages eleven to nineteen. Longitudinal bone growth continues until puberty, at which time the epiphyseal plates close. This is particularly important in children and adolescents, as the greatest amount of bone density increase occurs between the teenage years and the twenties.[10, 11] Peak bone mass is achieved in the third decade of life.

Low bone density results in the increased risk of fractures, including stress fractures. Stress fractures commonly occur in the feet, lower legs, and back, but can occur anywhere. Complete fractures can occur with minimal trauma in those with lowered bone density. The most ominous fractures are osteoporotic hip fractures. Those with lower bone density have a much harder time healing from these fractures.

Mortality rates are higher in postmenopausal individuals with hip fractures in the face of osteoporosis.[12] This is especially concerning in adolescents with a low bone density as a result of low sex hormones. They will be living with low bone density for a much longer time compared to postmenopausal individuals.

Testosterone-based bodies (cisgender men, some transgender women, and nonbinary individuals) can get osteoporosis when their testosterone levels drop and may develop osteoporosis even faster than estrogen-based bodies.[13, 14]

Unfortunately, it takes about a year for any change to be visible on a repeat bone density test.[15] The Academy for Eating Disorders (AED) recommends obtaining a baseline bone density test in clients with an eating disorder and repeating as necessary per physician recommendation to evaluate progress.

Common symptoms of low bone density seen in people with eating disorders are:

- Chronic bone or joint pain*
- Loss of menstrual cycle without pregnancy*
- Delay of menstrual cycle*
- Stress fractures*

Physician notification and involvement strongly advised.

Chemical Stew

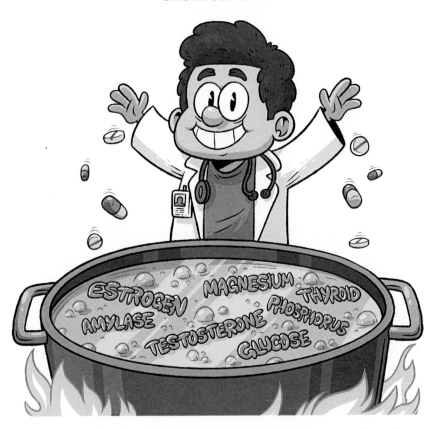

It is clear that eating disorders and malnutrition significantly impact the well-being of the body. The blood tests listed below are useful in the assessment of nutritional status caused by eating disorders. (The Medical Care Standards Guide written by the Academy for Eating Disorders, *Eating Disorders: A Guide to Medical Care*, is another excellent resource.)

Amylase—Levels may be increased in those who are purging (this is not always a specific test, however).

Bicarbonate—Will be elevated in individuals misusing diuretics and purging; will be lowered in individuals who misuse laxatives and have diarrhea.

Blood Urea Nitrogen—Levels are often low in individuals consuming very little protein.

Calcium—Levels are often low with abnormal levels of parathyroid hormone. Can also see low calcium levels in malnutrition and malabsorption syndromes. Normal calcium levels are not indicative of bone density.

Cholesterol—Elevated cholesterol is ironically seen in individuals with severe malnutrition and anorexia nervosa, because their bodies are unable to metabolize cholesterol like in a healthy person. Elevated cholesterol can be seen in individuals with binge-eating disorder.

Complete Blood Count (CBC):

> *Red Blood Cell Count*—Lowered in individuals with anorexia nervosa and malnutrition due to bone marrow suppression.

> *White Blood Count*—Lowered in individuals with anorexia nervosa and malnutrition due to bone marrow suppression.

> *Platelets*—Lowered due to malnutrition.

Creatinine—Levels are often lower in individuals with malnutrition, and correlate with abnormal kidney function.

Estradiol—Low in malnourished individuals. Leads to decreased bone density, decreased sexual desire, decreased ability to get pregnant, and irregular or absent menstrual periods.

Glucose—If low, can lead to "brain fog," sluggish memory, problems focusing or staying on track, light-headedness, serious cognitive dysfunction, fainting, incoordination, and possibly seizures and death.

Hemoglobin A1c—Represents a three-month average of serum glucose.

Liver Function Tests—Includes AST and ALT. Can be abnormal with drug and alcohol abuse, hepatitis, and starvation.

Magnesium—Low levels seen in malnutrition. Signs of magnesium deficiency include the loss of appetite, nausea, vomiting, fatigue, muscle cramps, and abnormal heart rate.

Phosphorus—Low levels seen in malnutrition. Also seen in rapid refeeding. Symptoms of phosphorus deficiency include confusion, altered mental status, muscle weakness, and fatigue.

Potassium—Lowered levels seen with bulimia nervosa due to self-induced vomiting/purging, and with diuretic or laxative misuse. Low levels generally not seen in anorexia nervosa unless engaging in above behaviors.

Testosterone—Low due to malnutrition.

Thyroid function test (T3, T4, and TSH)—Low levels seen as a result of malnutrition. Adequate nutrition, without the need for thyroid medication, can usually normalize these levels.

Other useful tests are:

Urinalysis—Can show evidence of kidney problems or dehydration. Specific gravity will be high in dehydration. Specific gravity will be low with water-loading.

EKG/ECG—Detects cardiac issues.

Blood Pressure/Pulse—A significant difference in blood pressure and pulse going from lying down to sitting can signal malnutrition and dehydration.

Temperature—Often lower than 98.6 degrees Fahrenheit in an individual with malnutrition.

Bone Density—Assesses degree of bone loss as a result of malnutrition.

The following screening questions can also be helpful in assessing for an eating disorder:

- I have thrown up at least once recently.
- I have taken some laxatives recently.
- I have taken stuff to make me throw up.
- I have taken some water pills recently.
- I have taken some other stuff that I would rather not talk about.
- I often drink enough alcohol to get drunk.

- I have had thoughts about killing myself recently.
- I have hurt myself by cutting, scratching, burning, or other forms of self-inflicted injury.
- I currently have these symptoms:
    - Feeling cold much of the time
    - Fingers or toes turn blue at times
    - "Hot flashes" or sweating not related to exercise
    - Dizziness or feeling like I'm going to pass out
    - Bruises
    - Dry mouth
    - Sudden fast heartbeat
    - My heart "skips beats" or "jumps" at times
    - Chest pain
    - Shortness of breath or trouble breathing
    - Difficulty concentrating
    - Difficulty with memory
    - Falling asleep or extreme fatigue during the daytime (e.g. at school or work)
    - Trouble falling or staying asleep at night
    - Loss or irregular menstrual periods
    - Thinning hair
    - Constipation or difficulty having a bowel movement
    - Swelling in my hands or feet
    - Stomach pain
    - Blood with vomiting or in stools
    - Throwing up something that looks like coffee grounds
    - Bone or joint pain
- About how many calories a day have you been eating for the last week?
- About how much fluid have you consumed in the last day?
- How much caffeine do you usually consume?
- Do you feel a need to exercise every day regardless of the circumstances?
- Do you exercise to "make up" for something you ate?
- Do you exercise even if you are injured?

Consider this analogy: If you had a fine European automobile and needed to replace its transmission, would you replace it? Or would you ask the mechanic to tweak the breaks, muffler, and steering wheel to compensate for the nonfunctioning transmission?

As shown in this chapter, all the organs of the body are impacted by malnutrition. The body's ability to temporarily compensate for these deficiencies will not prevent long-term damage.

Chapter 7 Notes

1. Elissa Rosen, "Health Myths of the Female Athlete, Myth 4: Bradycardia," Gaudiani Clinic, June 26, 2019, www.gaudianiclinic.com/gaudiani-clinic-blog/2019/6/25/health-myths-of-the-female-athlete-myth4-bradycardia-is-a-sign-of-good-fitness.

2. G. Frank, "Advances from neuroimaging studies in eating disorders," *CNS Spectrums* 20, no. 4 (August 2015): 391–400.

3. G. Frank, "Advances from neuroimaging studies."

4. Graham A. MacGregor et al., "Rebound Sodium and Water Retention Occurs When Diuretic Treatment Is Stopped," *British Medical Journal* 316, no. 7,131 (February 1998): 628.

5. Daniel S. Oh et al., "Pathophysiology and treatment of Barrett's esophagus," *World Journal of Gastroenterology* 16, no. 30 (August 2010): 3762–3772.

6. The terms estrogen-based bodies and testosterone-based bodies with their explanations are explained by Andrew Sage Mendez-McLeish.

7. S. Faubio et al., "Sexual Dysfunction in Women: A Practical Approach," *American Family Physician* 92, no. 4 (August 2015): 281–288.

8. R. Petering et al., "Testosterone Therapy: Review of Clinical Applications," *American Family Physician* 96, no. 7 (October 2017): 441–449.

9. L. Kalm et al., "They Starved So That Others Be Better Fed: Remembering Ancel Keys and the Minnesota Experiment," *The Journal of Nutrition* 135, no. 6 (June 2005): 1347–1352.

10. M. Misra, N. H. Golden, and D. K. Katzman, "State-of-the-art systematic review of bone disease in anorexia nervosa," *International Journal of Eating Disorders* 49, no. 3 (March 2016): 276–292.

11. S. Faubio, "Sexual Dysfunction in Women."

12. W. C. Hayes et al., "Impact near the hip dominates fracture risk in elderly nursing home residents who fall," *Calcified Tissue International* 52, no. 3 (March 1993): 192–198.

13. NIH Osteoporosis and Related Bone Diseases National Resource Center, "Osteoporosis Overview," National Institutes of Health, last reviewed October 2018, https://www.bones.nih.gov/health-info/bone/osteoporosis/overview.

14. Robert A. Adler, "Osteoporosis in men: a review," *Bone Research* 2 (April 2014). Published online.

15. J. Kling et al., "Osteoporosis Prevention, Screening, and Treatment: A Review," *Journal of Women's Health* 23, no. 7 (July 2014): 563–572.

PART III

THE BIG MACRO-FUEL
FOR YOUR MIND, BODY, AND SOUL

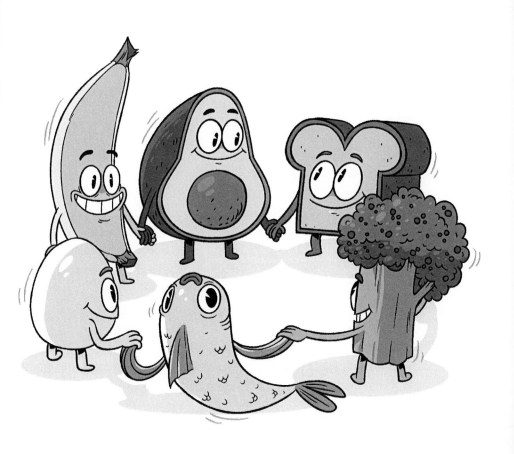

Consider any machine or piece of technology you've ever used. Vehicles, airplanes, cell phones, computers, cameras. As their inventors pondered their very existence, each faced answering a very important question: how will they run? From fuel to electricity to solar power, each of these pieces of technology needs an energy source to perform their functions.

The body is another amazing machine, and it also requires a power source to fuel its every action. In that sense, food is the answer.

There is no shortage of mixed messages in our society regarding what, when, and how much to eat. As a result, people struggle to feel satisfied, happy, or at ease in listening to, and trusting, their bodies. The unfortunate truth is that most of these unfounded and dangerous messages are spread only to further diet culture and, therefore, bolster consumerism.

Individuals with eating disorders often internalize these messages and transform them into a variety of food rules, following them as if they were law, to the detriment of their minds, bodies, and lives.

That doesn't have to be the case. It is possible to get out from under the thumb of an eating disorder or diet culture if only we become more educated in separating fact from fiction around the beliefs we learn from diet culture.

The next few chapters will support the reader in doing just that, stripping away the media messages and debunking myths and falsehoods that are pervasive in diet culture. If you are striving to relearn how to eat, become better connected with your body, and be more conscious of how various foods feel in your body, the information in these chapters will be invaluable to you. We will explore the basics of what fuels the extraordinary bodies that carry us through our lives—macronutrients.

Macronutrients are the three main elements of food: carbohydrates, proteins, and fats.

You may think you know the function and purpose of each of these, but it is likely these chapters will open your eyes to the incredible importance of these elements and how they support our bodies, our minds, and life itself. The purpose of these chapters is to help you feel empowered to make food selections that allow you to listen to your body and the wisdom that it possesses without having doubts, guilt, or shame.

CHAPTER 8

THE CARB CONUNDRUM: YOUR BRAIN'S BEST FRIEND

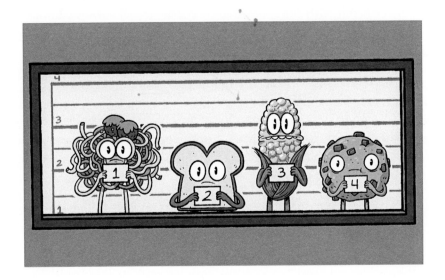

Carbs. Some might consider them a four-letter word. But the truth is that carbohydrates, like proteins and fats, play a crucial role in your overall health and well-being. As much as trendy diets may tell you to eliminate or reduce your carb intake, carbs are essential to nourishing your body and keeping you in good health. For those recovering from an eating disorder, there will likely be a time when your family member, therapist, or dietitian will suggest something very scary to you: reintroducing carbohydrates into your diet.

Our society has deemed carbohydrates to be evil, dangerous, and undesirable. However, the truth is that the benefits of carbohydrates are invaluable in the human body, meaning you absolutely need to include them in your healthy eating habits.

Putting it simply, carbohydrates are what I like to describe as the gasoline that fuels your car. In essence, they provide us with the thing necessary for living a happy and joyful life: energy.

Having a basic understanding of the importance of carbohydrates, and their positive impact on the body and mind, can help debunk untrue societal stigmas, and make the thought of consuming them less scary.

Let's begin with the understanding that not all carbohydrates are the same. In fact, there are two different types that serve important functions.

The first type of carbohydrates is complex carbohydrates. These are the carbohydrates found in cereal, rice, pasta, crackers, corn, peas, yams, potatoes, beans, non-starchy vegetables, and possibly the most well-known carbohydrate: bread! Long chains of glucose molecules make up complex carbohydrates. They provide a slow and steady re-lease of fuel into the bloodstream, as the bonds (the long chain of sugar units) take longer to break apart, and thus take longer to absorb. This type of carbohydrate takes longer to break down into sugar, also known as glucose, and provides fiber and water helping you to feel full. Complex carbohydrates also provide the body with important vitamins and minerals. The benefit of eating complex carbohydrates is that they can help stabilize blood sugar and mood, help us feel full, and help reduce cravings, fatigue, and/or headaches.

Simple carbohydrates are the other form of carbohydrates, and have developed a reputation just as negative as complex carbohydrates. Many people are not aware of the products they consume which are simple carbohydrates. These include fresh and dried fruit, fruit juice, milk, dairy products (including nondairy yogurts and nondairy milk made from rice, almond, flax, and coconut), desserts, baked goods, candy, sodas, and mixed alcoholic beverages. Simple carbohydrates consist of shorter glucose chains than complex carbohydrates, and therefore break down faster and enter the bloodstream quicker. This can cause blood sugar to spike and then drop, as the pancreas releases the hormone insulin to help the glucose enter the cells. Once glucose enters the cells, sugar levels in the blood begin to decrease. If blood sugar is not maintained by eating at regular intervals, the pancreas will release a different hormone called glucagon. Glucagon signals the liver to release stored sugar to help bring blood-sugar levels back up to normal. The actions of insulin and glucagon guarantee that cells throughout the body and brain maintain a consistent level of blood sugar. Rapid drops in blood sugar due to the action of insulin after eating simple carbohydrates can impact mood and cause individuals to become hungry soon after eating.

Another distinguishing factor is whether a carbohydrate contains fiber. Carbohydrates that contain fiber take longer to metabolize. The fiber, vitamins, and minerals in simple carbohydrates are removed during the refining process, and these foods are not as efficient in keeping blood sugar stable. Therefore, fiber-containing carbohydrates tend to fill us up sooner, leave us feeling full longer, and help keep our blood sugar and mood stable better than carbohydrates without fiber.

Whether simple or complex, carbohydrates are the number-one fuel used by our brain, and the number-one macronutrient required by our body. As a result, professionals recommend that carbohydrates make up 45 to 65 percent of our daily food intake. Since our brain cannot store glucose, effective brain functioning depends on the regular intake of carbohydrates so that the brain does not become fuel (glucose) deprived.

Inadequate carbohydrate intake can cause our behavior to change, and make us become irritable, tired, more emotional, unable to focus, to make irrational decisions, have brain fog, and become obsessed about food.

Carbohydrates are also required to make serotonin, a neurotransmitter that allows us to feel calm and relaxed. This is another way inadequate carbohydrate intake can impact our emotional well-being, and increase feelings of anxiety, including anxiety around food.

Carbohydrates, because of their fiber content, also play an important role in bowel movement regularity.

Our brain chemistry becomes altered when we are not consuming sufficient amounts of carbohydrates. Starvation can cause a hormone in our brain known as neuropeptide Y (NPY) to remain consistently elevated. In a person who doesn't have a dieting history or an eating disorder history, NPY levels will go down after eating, as is the normal process of this hormone. However, in an individual with an eating disorder, or in someone who often goes on and off diets, the elevated NPY levels do not come down the way they are supposed to. This elevated NPY level leads to having chronic thoughts about food and increasing cravings for carbohydrates, increasing the likelihood of binging.

Luckily, with adequate carbohydrate intake, it is possible to retrain the NPY hormone to perform as it once did.

Every cell in our body requires glucose throughout the entire day, including during sleep cycles. During the hours of sleep when we are not consuming carbohydrates, our body will pull glucose from the liver. In case there is not adequate glucose stored in the liver, glucose is created from the protein in our muscles in a process known as gluconeogenesis. It is thanks to this bodily process that we do not go braindead when we are asleep. Depriving our body of carbohydrates, and therefore glucose, can lead to inadequate stores to pull from, which can result in many health risks.

Just as a car cannot run without sufficient gasoline, our body cannot function long-term without carbohydrates and the vitamins, nutrients, and minerals they provide.

When we are struggling with an eating disorder, it is very common to have food rules that almost always include avoidance of various forms of carbohydrates. As you can see, this is a dangerous practice. We cannot demonize or single out any nutrient for being "good" or "bad," since nutrients do not work alone; instead, they work synergistically with the other nutrients in our food supply. In fact, labelling any nutrient as "good" or "bad" is dangerous and useless; food choices should not be given a moral value. Eating should be about pleasure, building connection, and having fun; food rules only take away from this.

The disdain and fear of eating carbohydrates are largely due to false diet culture messages about carbohydrates causing bloating and weight gain. Untrue! When we restrict carbohydrates or any food,

the gastrointestinal tract becomes malnourished. Malnutrition causes the stomach and intestines to slow down, leading to gastroparesis.
Gastrointestinal motility is delayed, and the individual may have a
more difficult time digesting food, which leads to feelings of being
bloated. (It is important to note that intestinal paralysis can occur with
chronic stimulant laxative abuse.) The pad of fat that protects the duodenum (part of the small intestine) shrinks due to malnutrition; this
causes the duodenum to be compressed between the abdominal aorta
and the overlying superior mesenteric artery. This is called SMA syndrome (superior mesenteric artery syndrome), and can be life-threatening. The perception that carbohydrates should be avoided therefore
becomes dangerous, because cutting carbohydrates out of one's diet
disrupts all of the systems mentioned above.

I ask my clients, "How often do you wake up in the middle of the
night in a cold sweat?" Many find themselves experiencing this symptom, despite not having exercised, feeling ill, or experiencing meno-
pause. This can be a result of insufficient carbohydrate intake, which
then results in hypoglycemia (low blood sugar), leading to night sweats.

By working with a nutrition therapist who specializes in eating disorders, we are able to help add carbohydrates back into one's diet. The
role of these nutrition therapists is to combat false diet culture messages
by explaining the function of these foods, as well as support the client
through their fear and ambivalence about any new food. The nutrition
therapist is necessary to help the client increase what they identify as
"safe foods" and decrease what they consider "fear foods." The nutrition therapist is invaluable in supporting the individual during this
scary and overwhelming time.

The vitamins, minerals, and nutrients found in carbohydrates cannot simply be replaced by other types of foods, making consuming carbohydrates critical to the optimal functioning of the body and mind.
It's as if your car needed gasoline, but you gave it motor oil instead.

As one introduces carbohydrates back into their diet, they will be
going against the food rules they had previously risked their lives following. As such, the voice of their eating disorder will become louder,
as its "dying" protest doesn't want the individual to succeed. To fight

this voice, the individual must push forward with their recovery-focused behaviors, including the initiation of carbohydrates back into the diet.

Doing the opposite of what we know and have lived for sometimes requires more energy and focus. Thus, during this time in recovery, I recommend clients become "the person they have never had the courage to be." Over time, they will discover they are that person. Eventually, these new behaviors will feel like second nature and become a habit. Until then, I encourage them to be kind, empathic, and nurturing toward themselves as they navigate these challenging changes.

CHAPTER 9

PROTEIN: TOO MUCH OR TOO LITTLE?

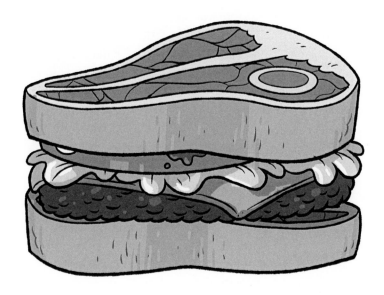

We've had our fill, pun intended, of carbohydrates in the last chapter. So let's shift to a new topic: protein. Unlike carbohydrates, many believe proteins to be "safe" per the trendy "diet du jour." As individuals have decreased the amount of carbohydrates in their diet based on false fear, they have increased their intake of proteins.

Carbohydrates and proteins are not interchangeable. Each serves a different purpose, and has its own important bodily function. Just as carbohydrates are necessary and important for the brain, proteins are very critical to the entire functioning of the body.

Proteins are made of various amino acids. Some of these amino acids are essential, meaning we must get them from our food. Others are called nonessential, because our body is able to make them. Protein plays many important roles in our body. For example, protein is essential for the growth and repair of all the cells in our body. It is the primary building block of muscle, skin, hair, nails, and bone. Without adequate protein intake, one can experience diminished bone, skin, hair, and poor muscle maintenance and development. This can present as muscle wasting, the loss of skeletal muscle and heart muscle, resulting in inadequate heart function. Protein is also needed for making neurotransmitters, various hormones, red and white blood cells, and antibodies. Therefore, inadequate protein intake can result in changes in the function of the brain and hormones, as well as a reduction in immunity. Protein foods contain an array of vitamins (vitamins B6, B12, niacin, thiamin, and riboflavin) and minerals (iron, zinc, and magnesium).

Protein can be found in animal-based foods, such as poultry, red meat, eggs, or dairy. A good rule of thumb is that anything with a face is animal-based protein. Protein can also be found in plant-based foods, such as soybeans, tofu, edamame, tempeh, seitan, veggie burgers, dried beans, nuts, seeds, and nut butters.

Let's take a little detour and talk about hunger. Often, people are aware of the "typical" signs of hunger in the body: a growling stomach, or an empty feeling in the stomach. At other times, people are not in touch with their hunger signals or choose to ignore them. Energy levels, mood, and sleep can all be influenced by hunger. Feeling tired can be a sign of hunger. Individuals may not be aware that sometimes low energy is a sign of hunger too. It doesn't always have to be felt in our belly. Extreme examples of hunger can be a headache or a hazy, light-headed feeling. In addition, people can experience a lack of concentration, a change in mood, and fatigue. If hunger consistently goes unacknowledged, these signs can come to feel normal. Learning the signs of hunger is an important skill to attain.

Feelings of hunger are impacted by two hormones: ghrelin and leptin. Ghrelin acts to increase our appetite and stimulate feelings of hunger. Ghrelin also increases the gastric enzyme production of neuropeptide Y (NPY). NPY influences our appetite and food choices.

Neuropeptide Y plays a role in sleep regulation as well. When our sleep is sporadic, these hormones can be dysregulated. Leptin, on the other hand, influences our satiety and fullness levels.

Protein takes three to four hours to digest. Eating protein tends to increase levels of satiety and satisfaction. Recently, a study published in the Academy of Nutrition and Dietetics showed that consuming more protein may increase fullness levels when compared to consuming less protein, as protein activates the satiety hormone leptin.[1]

The Pros and Cons of Protein

As mentioned above, the cultural trend is that protein is "in" and carbohydrates are "out." Many people overconsume protein in an attempt to develop more muscle. They are misinformed. Our body composition is determined by more than just protein intake. It is influenced by genetics, movement, and dieting history.

Another belief that holds little scientific evidence is the fear that eating too much protein can result in the kidneys' working overtime, and leading to long-term kidney damage. Research suggests that this may be the case only if one has a preexisting kidney condition.[2]

There is also concern that consuming too much animal-based protein will increase the risk for heart disease because of elevated cholesterol levels from the saturated fat content. Studies are inconclusive on the effects of protein intake and heart disease. Evidence supports following plant-based dietary patterns that emphasize protein-rich plant foods, and including some animal-based protein as well.

There is also concern that consuming too much animal-based protein can be detrimental to bone health. Studies reveal that there are no harmful effects on bone density with higher amounts of protein intake.[3, 4]

On the flip side, there are consequences to underconsumption of protein too. When individuals have a suboptimal amount of protein in their diet, they are more likely to feel tired, hungry, or "hangry," despite having just had a meal. This is probably due to the impact of leptin levels.[5]

There is a minimum requirement for protein intake so that our organs and tissues work properly.[6] Protein needs vary per person based on age, gender, and activity levels. On average, the recommended intake amount is 0.8 grams of protein per kilogram of body weight. When our bodies are fed adequate protein, we maintain adequate visceral and somatic protein stores, produce adequate neurotransmitters, hormones, and other protein-based compounds. Extreme cases of inadequate protein (and calorie) intake can lead to autophagy. This is when our protein/muscle stores waste away, and we "eat away" at our own organs in order to stay alive.

The muscle breakdown stated above, as well as the accompanying fat loss caused by starvation, can lead to liver failure. Laboratory testing would show elevated liver enzymes (AST and ALT), and physical examination would show edema (fluid retention) in the lower extremities: legs, feet, and/or ankles.

The truth is, either way you slice it, protein consumption must be balanced.

In my practice, I help clients see the correlation between their restrictive eating and physical symptoms. Often, they can see that their undernutrition is the cause of their fatigue, skin texture changes, thinning hair, or hair loss. Other symptoms can be dry scalp, muscle aches, waking up in a cold sweat, feeling cold all the time, and dental problems. Furthermore, adequate food intake is important in achieving and maintaining sufficient bone mass, as well as preventing osteoporosis. Undereating can also lead to being sick frequently due to a compromised immune system.

Overall, protein is an important nutrient for achieving stability in our health and enabling us to feel satisfaction from eating. Learning to balance it with other food groups will result in making more confident food choices.

Chapter 9 Notes

1. Jaapna Dhillon, "The Effects of Increased Protein Intake on Fullness: A Meta-Analysis and Its Limitations," *Journal of the Academy of Nutrition and Dietetics* 116, no. 6 (July 2015): 968–983.

2. Michaela Devries, "Changes in Kidney Function Do Not Differ between Healthy Adults Consuming Higher- Compared with Lower- or Normal-Protein Diets: A Systematic Review and Meta-Analysis," *The Journal of Nutrition* 148, no. 11 (November 2018): 1760–1775.

3. S. Sahni et al., "Dietary approaches for bone health: lessons from the Framingham Osteoporosis Study," *Current Osteoporosis Report* 13, no. 4 (August 2015): 245–255.

4. M. M. Shams-White et al., "Dietary protein and bone health: a systematic review and meta-analysis from the National Osteoporosis Foundation," *American Journal of Clinical Nutrition* 105, no. 6 (June 2017): 1528–1543.

5. P. Morrell and S. Fiszman, "Revisiting the role of protein-induced satiation and satiety," *Food Hydrocolloids* 68 (July 2017): 199–210.

6. National Research Council (US) Subcommittee on the Tenth Edition of the Recommended Dietary Allowances, "Protein and Amino Acids," chap. 6 in *Recommended Dietary Allowances: 10th Edition* (Washington, DC: National Academies Press, 1989).

CHAPTER 10

FAT: A FORGOTTEN FRIEND

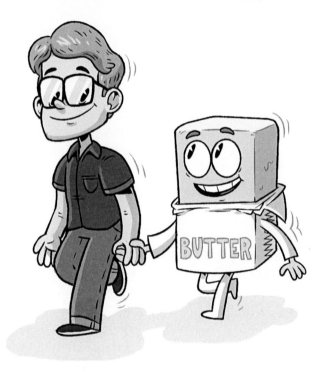

Poor fat. Fat is the most judged of all the macronutrients. Negative and stigmatizing messages around eating fat, having fat, or being fat abound in our society.

Separating misconceptions from the truth about fat may be challenging, but I'm going to do just that in this chapter. I am going to debunk myths and spread truths. Open your mind, say goodbye to diet culture lies, and give fat a chance.

Fat Is Your Friend

Fat serves two main purposes: it maintains proper body function, and it helps us achieve satisfaction from food.

The fat in our body is known as adipose tissue. We all have adipose tissue, whether we want it or not. And we should all want it, because body fat plays numerous important roles in the proper functioning of our bodies.

We live in a fat-phobic culture that views having body fat as negative and harmful, whereas the real danger exists in not having enough body fat.

Body fat plays the important role of maintaining our body temperature. When we lack adequate body fat, we can feel cold, or vacillate between feeling hot, warm, and cold. There is no consistency in the management of our body temperature. Clients sometimes tell me that their core body temperature doesn't change, but their hands, toes, and nose get cold. Think of body fat as your built-in thermostat, helping you to stabilize your body temperature as needed.

Adequate body fat stores, as mentioned before, allow us to have more sustained energy. This includes the energy needed for movement. Movement should not be focused on "burning calories." There's no need to punish yourself if you are not able to fit it in your schedule, and there is no need to alter food intake with regard to such movement, or lack thereof.

When we include fat in our meals, we tend to not get hungry as fast after a meal, thus not be preoccupied with thoughts of food in between meals.

Body fat is also necessary for the proper development of sex hormones; it impacts ovulation in women, and supports the induction of labor for women who are pregnant.

Furthermore, fat intake affects the formation of prostaglandins, which play a role in inflammation in the body, enabling wound healing, for example. In addition, eating fat helps with the management of blood sugar too.

In summary, body fat is necessary for the proper functioning of our bodies. Sadly, these crucial functions are never talked about in the messages disseminated by diet culture. Becoming informed and educated about the purpose of body fat is important for all people, including our healthcare providers.

So how does our body determine how much body fat it needs? There are two critical aspects to consider: one is a "set point" theory, and the other is the effect of activity level and environment. A well-known study, showing how weight is influenced by genetics, was conducted by Albert Stunkard, MD, and colleagues. They looked at twins separated at birth and brought up separately.[1, 2] They found that even when raised separately, the body weight of the twins closely matched each other. They concluded, "Genetic influences on body-mass index are substantial, whereas the childhood environment has little or no influence."[3] Another example is the research done by James Hill, PhD. His research demonstrates that multiple small changes in environmental factors may have an influence on body fat, such as eating behavior, daily activity, and sleep.

In addition, the body has mechanisms to resist changes in body fat stores, which can offset mathematical expectations based on calorie intake calculations. Leibel and colleagues showed that even when subjects were overfed, weight gain was resisted by increasing metabolic rate. Conversely, on a calorie-restricted meal plan, metabolic rate was decreased and weight loss was resisted.[4] These studies suggest that mechanisms beyond a person's voluntary control regulate energy stores, and these mechanisms can make it easier or harder for different individuals to change their body weight.

It would be great to have all healthcare providers be weight-inclusive providers who understand the facts about what contributes to body composition, instead of blindly applying the mathematical equation "calories in must equal calories out."

Our bodies are not math equations. The Vermont prisoner study validates this fact. In this study, subjects were overfed for eighty-four days. Twin participants received an additional one thousand calories per day. Based on traditional calculations, the predicted weight increase was to be twenty-four pounds. The results, however, showed a range of weight gain from nine to thirty pounds. This is a good example demonstrating that traditional equations are not good predictors of body weight change. Rather, it is a blend of genetics, physiology, hormones, dieting history, and our body's preferred "set point" weight that impacts body weight outcomes.[5]

Fat Is Delicious

Dietary fat in our food not only adds taste, flavor, and texture, but it also helps us feel satiated. Dietary fat intake also helps with absorption of important vitamins. A recent study found evidence to support that fat is crucial to the absorption of seven different micronutrients: four carotenoids (alpha and beta carotene, lutein, and lycopene) and vitamins A, D, E, and K (fat-soluble vitamins).[6]

Dietary fats come in two forms: saturated and unsaturated fats.

Saturated fats are most often, but not always, animal-based and solid at room temperature. They are any fat that is on meat, poultry, dairy products, egg yolks, creamy salad dressings, chocolate, ice cream, cookies, and baked goods. There are a few plant-sourced saturated fats as well. These are coconut oil, palm and palm kernel oil, palm fruit, cocoa butter, and cottonseed oil. There is some evidence that medium chain triglycerides (MCTs) found in coconut and palm oil (which contain lauric acid) can be beneficial for memory.[7] (Interestingly, breast milk naturally contains lauric acid too.)

Unsaturated fats are plant-based and liquid at room temperature. Unsaturated fats are divided into smaller categories: monounsaturated and polyunsaturated fats. Monounsaturated fats are found in various forms of nuts and their oils, such as olive, avocado, peanuts, and cashews. Polyunsaturated fats are also found in nuts and oils, such as in almonds and almond oil, walnuts and walnut oil, pecans, sunflower oil, safflower oil, flaxseeds, flaxseed meal, chia and hemp hearts, and corn oil.

The most well-known type of polyunsaturated fat is omega-3 fatty acids. The three types of omega-3 fatty acids are eicosapentaenoic acid (EPA), docosahexaenoic acid (DHA), and alpha linolenic acid (ALA). Alpha linolenic acid is one of two essential fatty acids (the other being alpha linoleic acid, which is an omega-6 fatty acid). This means that we must eat them in our food, because our bodies are not able to make them. Other food sources that provide omega-3 fatty acids include cold-water fish such as salmon, trout, mackerel, herring, and sardines. There are also foods that are fortified with omega-3s such as eggs, juices, and nondairy beverages such as soy milk, flax milk, and hemp milk, as well as infant formulas. There are many benefits of omega-3 fatty acids: they help with depression, anxiety, and other mood disorders; and help with sleeping difficulties. Omega-3 fatty acids are a key component in fetal brain development during pregnancy, and during the beginning stages of life. Omega-3 fatty acids are also important for heart health.

The Functions of Fat

Fats are our body's secondary fuel source (carbohydrates being the primary fuel source).

Ingesting fat is necessary to supply our bodies with the essential fatty acids it is unable to produce on its own. These fats are imperative and essential for healthy skin, hair, and nails, as well as brain development in utero. Fats are also necessary for temperature regulation, organ protection and padding, and are a key player in reproductive hormone levels and menstruation. Furthermore, fat promotes flexibility in our body by lubricating our joints. Essentially, without fats, our bodies dry up and we begin to resemble the scarecrow from *The Wizard of Oz*!

Fats are key to absorbing and transporting the fat-soluble vitamins—vitamins A, D, E, and K—throughout the body. Without adequate fat ingestion, we would not absorb these vitamins. Vitamin A is important for growth and bone development, reproduction, vision, and skin health. Vitamin D, the sunshine vitamin, is a key player in the maintenance of healthy bones. It helps maintain our calcium levels as well as our phosphorous levels. No one wants their bones to turn into Swiss cheese, do they? Vitamin E is an antioxidant. It protects the body's tissues from free radical damage. Lastly, vitamin K is important for blood clotting and helps to regulate blood calcium levels.

Fat is also necessary for the structure and function of all the cells in our nervous system. Our brain is made up of approximately 60 percent fat, and the fat is necessary for the brain to function optimally. Fat is critical for the development of neurotransmitters and hormones in our body.

When eating, it is important to have fat for flavor, taste, satiety, and satisfaction. I like to say that fat adds joy, what I call "vitamin J," to meals. It is not a fun experience to eat and then be preoccupied with when the next meal will be, due to a lack of fat in the meal. Dietary fat promotes satisfaction from food, and keeps us fuller longer. People who don't consume enough fat don't feel as satisfied with their meals, which as The Rolling Stones would say, "Can't Get No Satisfaction."

Many clients avoid eating fat to prevent elevated cholesterol levels. In fact, cholesterol levels can actually be falsely elevated when underweight and inadequately nourished. As such, elevated cholesterol readings are common in individuals struggling with anorexia nervosa because of an increase in low-density lipoproteins (LDL), because their bodies are unable to metabolize cholesterol normally.

Did you know that 5 percent of our total blood cholesterol level is attributed to dietary intake, and the remaining 95 percent is produced by our body? When we are in a state of stress, for example, our cortisol levels increase. This causes our body to overproduce cholesterol, and has nothing to do with the ingestion of fat. Managing stress and eating enough, then, may be a better way to manage cholesterol levels, rather than creating more "food rules" and following a low-cholesterol, low-fat diet.[8, 9]

Who knew something as ridiculed and judged as fat was crucial to so many important bodily functions? Diet culture won't tell you the truth. By sending the message that eating fat will "make you fat," diet culture promotes the "low-fat" and "fat-free" product market, driving up food costs for you. Conversely, promoters of "high-fat diets" will make you believe that eating only fat (and not carbohydrates) will have you living in a small body.

These rampant and harmful messages and misconceptions about fat impact the development of unhealthy food rules and disordered eating behaviors.

Individuals who struggle with eating disorder behaviors are often looking to gain a sense of control in their life. Having various rules about specific foods or food groups gives them a false sense of this control. Because of cultural misconceptions that fats are "bad," "harmful," or "not necessary," dietary fat has been cut out of diets, and body fat has become a popular body part to be altered, reduced, or cut out.

People with disordered eating beliefs or behaviors also often obtain their entire self-value from what they eat and their body size, shape, or weight. The ability to not eat fat, for example, gives them a sense of control and superiority. Is body size a good indicator of health? According to Jennifer L. Gaudiani, MD, CEDS, FAED, author of *Sick Enough: A Guide to the Medical Complications of Eating Disorders,* "The individual may look 'normal' because size does not indicate whether an individual may be 'sick enough.'"[10] If you are considering treatment, and find that your life is centered on what you will or will not eat, then you are "sick enough" and deserve treatment and help.

The longer food rules continue, the harder it makes it for individuals to remember what it felt like to function comfortably and optimally back when they were nourishing themselves fully. Although clients tell me they feel "fine" having cut out certain food groups from their diet, it is likely because they are not paying attention to the subtle negative changes their body is going through, which can lead to irreversible damage in the long term.

As scary as it may be for clients to lose their sense of control, it is important to teach them the benefits of reintroducing fear foods back into their diet. Only then, having felt the difference, can they appreciate the health costs of listening to the lies their eating disorder has told them.

Our culture perpetuates negative ideas about fat that make cutting it out of our lives seem harmless and easy. In reality, it is incredibly harmful because we would not be able to survive if we didn't have body fat or consume dietary fat. Fat's unfair reputation as unnecessary and harmful is unfounded. The truth is that fat adds flavor, texture, satisfaction, and fun to our food and to our lives!

Chapter 10 Notes

1. A. J. Stunkard et al., "The body-mass index of twins who have been reared apart," *New England Journal of Medicine* 322, no. 21 (May 1990):1483–1487.

2. A. J. Stunkard et al., "An adoption study of human obesity," *New England Journal of Medicine* 314, no. 4 (January 1986):193–198.

3. James Hill, "Understanding and Addressing the Epidemic of Obesity: An Energy Balance Perspective," *Endocrine Review* 27, no. 7 (December 2006): 750–761.

4. R. L. Leibel, M. Rosenbaum, and J. Hirsch, "Changes in energy expenditure resulting from altered body weight," *New England Journal of Medicine* 332, no. 10 (March 1995): 621–628.

5. L. B. Salans, E. S. Horton, and E. A. Sims, "Experimental obesity in man: cellular character of the adipose tissue," *Journal of Clinical Investigation* 50, no. 5 (May 1971):1005–1011.

6. W. White, "Iowa State University researcher finds further evidence that fats and oils help to unlock full nutritional benefits of veggies," Iowa State University News Service, October 9, 2017.

7. Candida Rebello et al., "Pilot feasibility and safety study examining the effect of medium chain triglyceride supplementation in subjects with mild cognitive impairment: A randomized controlled trial," *BBA Clinical Journal* 3 (June 2015): 123–125.

8. G. A. Soliman, "Dietary cholesterol and the lack of evidence in cardiovascular disease," *Nutrients* 10, no. 6 (June 2018): 780.

9. S. Gropper, J. Smith, and J. Groff, *Advanced Nutrition and Human Metabolism 5th edition* (Belmont, CA: Wadsworth Publishing, 2008), 166–167.

10. Jennifer L. Gaudiani, *Sick Enough: A Guide to the Medical Complications of Eating Disorders* (London: Routledge, 2018).

CHAPTER 11

WATER: FIND YOUR BALANCE

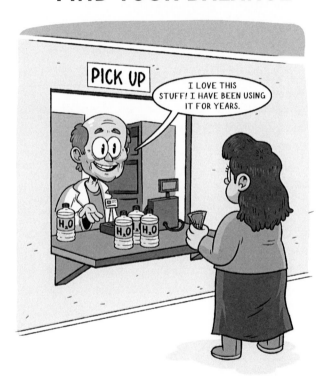

I cannot overstate the value of water to our mental and physical functioning, to our well-being, and to the world in general. Water has a tremendous number of functions, all relevant to the health of your body and the overall health of Planet Earth. It would be an understatement to say water is life, because it really is so much more. In this chapter, I will explore the importance of water to your body, and its role in your organs such as your brain and your heart. At the end of this chapter, I am confident you will recognize the incredible significance of this seemingly mundane miracle fluid.

Even since before scientists understood the complex inner workings of the body, water has been viewed as essential to the soul. This odorless, colorless liquid is seen not only as nourishing and replenishing, but also as cleansing—both physically and spiritually. Word of its importance spans time, geography, and culture.

Despite the slight differences that may exist between the cultural and religious understandings of the symbolism of water, most agree that water is representative of vitality. In fact, water is crucial to all of the internal processes of living that we may take for granted.[1]

Water is required for our body to accomplish all of the processes necessary for life, and therefore, up to 90 percent of our body weight is made up of water. In fact, the organs most crucial to life-giving factors such as breathing and blood flow contain predominantly water. The brain and heart are composed of 73 percent water, and the lungs are about 83 percent water. The skin contains about 64 percent water, muscles and kidneys contain 79 percent water, and bones consist of 31 percent water.[2, 3]

All bodily processes that require fluids—urination, perspiration, saliva formation, blood, lymphatic fluid, digestive juices, and teardrops—require water. Water helps our body with the absorption of nutrients and adequate digestion. Water is necessary to help prevent constipation, avoid headaches, fight illness and/or disease, and manage our body's temperature regulation.

Water also maintains our skin tone, and allows for our muscles to contract.[4] If we lack hydration, our muscles will be unable to contract and our skin tone will become "rubbery." If you were to pull someone's skin that was dehydrated or lacked enough water, you would notice a reduced elastic rebounding effect, taking longer for the skin to return to its original position.

So, water is important. Seems simple enough, right? But when it comes to eating disorders and nutrition, nothing is really simple. The truth is, just as eating can become disordered, so can drinking, and water often becomes a central factor in these disordered behaviors.

Many individuals who struggle with disordered eating alter their fluid intake, and they predominantly do so via a process known as "fluid loading." Fluid loading refers to an individual drinking too much liquid, done to mask hunger and result in a feeling of "fake fullness." In this process, liquids (water or other noncaloric beverages) are consumed in large amounts to reach maximum stomach capacity. However, since they are consuming no calories to feel satiated, this only results in a short-term feeling of "fullness," and bloating. Undernourished clients also falsely elevate their weight during checkups with their healthcare team through fluid loading.

An excess intake of water or noncaloric liquids will not result in satiation or nourishment, but will undoubtedly wreak havoc on the body. The body works hard to maintain electrolyte levels in the blood within a narrow range. The excess consumption of fluids can dilute these electrolytes (sodium, potassium, calcium, magnesium, chloride), leading to serious health consequences. Hyponatremia, or low blood levels of sodium, for example, can lead to confusion and disorientation. This phenomenon is appropriately referred to as water intoxication. Hypokalemia, or low potassium levels in the blood as a result of dilution, can mess with the rhythm of the heart, cause nausea, vomiting, or fainting. Hypocalcemia, or low blood calcium levels, can lead to irregular muscle contractions and cramping. Imbalanced and suboptimal levels of electrolytes can also result in epileptic seizures, and blood pressure becoming dangerously low.

The converse to overconsumption of fluid is dehydration, caused by an inadequate consumption of liquids, or the use of diuretics, laxatives, or medications that make you vomit (emetic drugs). Diuretics (also known as "water pills") increase urine output. Laxatives increase stool output (although this result can diminish over time as the bowels build a tolerance to the laxative). Some patients with an eating disorder abuse diuretics and laxatives and emetic drugs in an attempt to lose weight. This "weight loss," however, is caused by mostly water loss, or dehydration. Unfortunately the problem is compounded, because not only do these agents increase the excretion of fluid, but also of electrolytes, leaving the person with the above-stated consequences of low blood electrolytes. The misuse of diuretics, laxatives, and emetic agents can lead to many health consequences, among them kidney failure, a "lazy bowel" (a slowing of the bowels that leads to constipation and painful bowel movements as a result of the frequent use of laxatives), and in the case of syrup of ipecac, a torn esophagus.

Another diet tactic used by clients is the adherence to a low-carbohydrate diet. Interestingly, low-carbohydrate diets act as a diuretic by increasing the excretion of fluids and minerals, again leading to dehydration.

Dehydration can also be caused by simply not taking in enough liquids, for clients restrict fluids along with food. Dehydration has many signs because of all the bodily functions that require water. Dehydrated individuals may experience cramping or tingling in their arms, hands, legs, or feet; their skin may become clammy and pale; their eyes may become irritated and appear red or pink; and body temperature can become dysregulated.[5] Dehydration also affects mood and can result in instability, mood swings, and an inability to think rationally or engage in conversation. Brain function can also be impacted leading to fogginess, difficulty thinking, headaches, dizziness, and in extreme cases, vomiting. It is possible, though, for an individual to be dehydrated and not experience the above-mentioned symptoms. Dehydration can lead to diminished urine output and constipation. And it can also impact endurance and physical performance in exercise. Dehydration can decrease blood volume, lowering blood pressure and not allowing adequate blood to reach vital organs.

In order for the body to function optimally, then, it is important to avoid fluid overloading and engaging in behaviors that promote dehydration. This inevitably leads to the question, "How much fluid should be consumed per day?" The answer is the same annoying yet freeing answer given to any question about quantity with regard to food or beverage: it varies from person to person.

Think of your body as a plant. Consider all the different types of plants and the varying level of watering they need. How much water an individual needs to consume is based on numerous factors such as their activity level, the amount of sweat produced, the climate, the temperature, and the altitude. A number you are probably familiar with is the recommendation to drink eight eight-ounce glasses of fluid per day. This number is completely arbitrary, but is probably a good place to start. And as you become aware of what optimal hydration feels like to you, you can adjust this number accordingly.

Then perhaps the next question is, "What is the best fluid to drink?" Scientists will agree that water is the fluid of choice. However, there have been many "enhancers," in the form of drops added to water, introduced in the market to help water become more palatable. Since most of these enhancers contain artificial sweeteners and other chemicals, you are best off sticking to water. Decaffeinated tea and decaffeinated coffee will mostly provide the same benefit. And fruits and vegetables are naturally water-rich as well.

How about alkaline water? Alkaline water refers to water that has had its pH increased to higher than seven, which is the neutral pH of normal drinking water. Many health claims have been made about the benefits of drinking alkaline water. As of now, there is a lack of scientific research supporting these claims. The truth is, just like the body works hard to maintain electrolyte levels within a narrow range, the kidneys and lungs work hard to maintain pH within a narrow range too.

A word about caffeine. Although decaffeinated coffee can be used to meet some of one's daily fluid needs, coffee (or other caffeinated beverages) are often abused by patients with an eating disorder. Not only do caffeinated beverages have a mild diuretic, thus dehydrating, effect, they can also have an appetite-suppressant quality.[6] For some clients, it is easier to just drink fluids (preferably low-calorie ones) than to ingest solid food. For other clients, the opposite is true. Patients who consume large amounts of caffeinated beverages instead of water may require an electrolyte-replacement beverage, coconut water, or electrolyte chews. These products, because of their varied electrolyte and calorie content, are a better choice than salt tabs, which only contain sodium.

Again, if you think of your body as a plant, with water, it flourishes, without water, it dries up. If water equals life and vitality, lack of water equals destruction, depletion, and in the worst-case scenario, death. Find the sweet spot of hydration and nourishment, and allow yourself to blossom and flourish.

Chapter 11 Notes

1. Barry M. Popkin et al., "Water, Hydration and Health," *Nutrition Reviews* 68, no. 8 (August 2010): 439–458.

2. H. H. Mitchell et al., "The Chemical Composition of the Adult Human Body and Its Bearing on the Biochemistry of Growth," *Journal of Biological Chemistry* 158 (February 1945): 628.

3. US Geological Survey, "The Water in You: Water and the Human Body," US Department of the Interior, accessed December 17, 2019, https://www.usgs.gov/special-topic/water-science-school/science/water-you-water-and-human-body?qt-science_center_objects=0#qt-science_center_objects.

4. L. Palma et al., "Dietary water affects human skin hydration and biomechanics," *Clinical Cosmetic and Investigational Dermatology* 8 (August 2015): 413–421. Published online.

5. Popkin et al., "Water, Hydration and Health."

6. Division of Nutrition, Physical Activity, and Ob*sity and the National Center for Chronic Disease Prevention and Health Promotion, "Get the Facts: Drinking Water and Intake," Centers of Disease Control and Prevention, last reviewed August 9, 2016, https://www.cdc.gov/nutrition/data-statistics/plain-water-the-healthier-choice.html.

PART IV

THE ROAD TO RECOVERY: COMPASSION

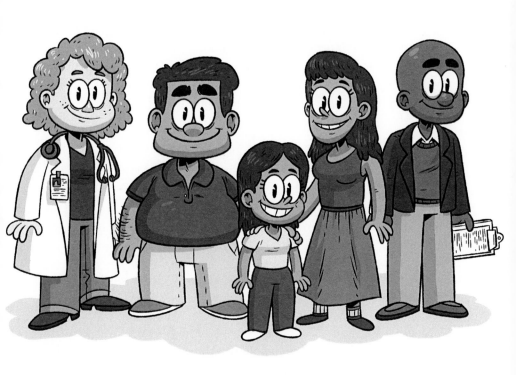

Just as compassion is an invaluable ingredient to humanity, it is a crucial part of eating disorder treatment and recovery. These remaining chapters will explore this concept of compassion in all of its facets— from the treatment team to loved ones to the self.

A compassionate treatment team is one that understands there is no shortcut on the road to recovery from an eating disorder. Patients will experience wrong turns, unplanned catastrophes, and moments that slow down or halt the journey toward a healthy life. It takes a lot of time for patients to experience the freedom from the mental, emotional, and physical drain of an eating disorder. But you will likely see strength, and a series of uncomfortable decisions on the part of the individual fighting. It is imperative that treatment team members are understanding and empathetic of this so that they can provide nonjudgmental and unconditional support and help the client exist in the most effective headspace for recovery.[1]

If you are not coming from a place of compassion when treating an individual with an eating disorder, it will show in the provided treatment. How? Well, it will make it harder for patients to open up in one of the most vulnerable times of their life. It is crucial that patients connect to you, and trust that you are there with them empathetically and withholding judgment. People with eating disorders already experience a tremendous amount of shame and judge themselves enough as it is. The addition of a judgmental treatment could be what deters them from continuing treatment or achieving recovery.

Compassion for the self is another key ingredient to recovery. It involves understanding that we cannot control everything or please everyone, and accepting that this is okay and does not signal a failure on our part. Learning how to say what you mean, while it may be scary and painful, is necessary in moving closer toward recovery.[2]

The "eating disorder voice" is possibly the largest barrier to saying what we mean and embracing self-love and compassion in recovery. Thus, it is vital that we clarify and explore what this voice is, where it comes from, and how it can rob us of self-love, self-identity, and compassion for the self. Perhaps most importantly, the reader will learn how to say goodbye to it and, instead, listen to their own intuition by learning to tune in to their own inner voice and acknowledging their feelings as real and normal with kindness, gentleness, nonjudgment, and self-compassion.

Finally, the reader will learn how to advocate and develop boundaries for oneself and communicate these to their loved ones openly and honestly, whether it be opening up about challenging thoughts or feelings in recovery, communicating a need to skip an event, or combatting a stigmatizing or judgmental statement.

If the previous parts of this book focused on the wreckage an eating disorder creates, the following chapters will look at restoration, exploring how to find your own inner voice, listen to it, and communicate that to your loved ones and treatment team as well as incorporating it into your new, free life.

You have spent enough time hating and fighting yourself, so let's look at how you can know and begin to like, or even love, yourself.

We have had enough talk about the breakdown. Let's work through the healing.

Part IV Introduction Notes

1. A. Macbeth et al., "Exploring compassion: A meta-analysis of the association between self-compassion and psychopathology," *Clinical Psychology Review* 32, no. 6 (August 2012): 545–552.

2. Kristen Neff, *Self-Compassion: The Proven Power of Being Kind to Yourself* (New York: HarperCollins, 2011).

CHAPTER 12

THE EATING DISORDER VOICE: WHO TO LISTEN TO?

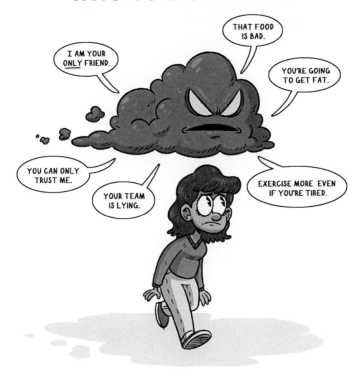

We all have an inner bully that makes us doubt ourselves, our worth, and our identity. This is the voice that tears us down as we strive to build ourselves up. For eating-disordered individuals, this voice is a crippling constant that often runs the show and encourages the perpetuation of unhealthy and harmful behaviors. But the voice is not the enemy; it has something to tell you.

Carolyn Costin, LMFT, CEDS, a renowned therapist specializing in eating disorders, was the first person to write about the eating disorder as a separate aspect of the self, an ego state that develops over time. She explains this concept in her books:

> I have found this voice to be universal in people who have eating disorders, and have come to regard it as the voice of the person's "Eating Disorder Self." It is not something outside of the person but more like an internal critic that develops over time. A large part of my work with eating disorder clients is helping them identify their "Eating Disorder Self" and then strengthen their Healthy Self, so it can challenge the eating disorder and get back in control. The goal is not to get rid of the Eating Disorder Self, but to learn how it is serving the person. The goal is to strengthen the Healthy Self to take over the job. The idea is to integrate the Eating Disorder Self and the Healthy Self so there is no longer a split, but one self love.[1]

We all have a "healthy self" we are born with. A variety of things can happen to a person that, combined with their genetic predisposition, can cause them to develop an eating disorder mindset that becomes like a separate personality. As this eating disorder self unfolds, it can take over the healthy self, muddling its wisdom. As mentioned above, the goal is not to get rid of the split-off eating disorder self, but to learn the purpose it is serving and then strengthen the person's healthy self so it can take over the job. The end result is the elimination of the eating disorder behaviors and integrating the split-off eating disorder self back into the core self so there is one whole person again.

When clients are engaged in this manner, it makes them feel much less threatened. You are not taking away their eating disorder self, but helping them discover its purpose and finding better ways to fulfill that purpose. This stance is invaluable in helping clients gain insight about their eating disorder, and eventually strengthen their healthy self so that they no longer need the eating disorder behaviors.

The stories I hear usually go something like this: Life was going well until a transition happened that made the client feel out of control. It was too scary or uncomfortable to talk to someone about, so the client chose to take things into their own hands—if they could just lose a little weight, become more fit, and eat a "cleaner diet," things would be so much more manageable. Yet despite being "healthier," the stressful situation wasn't resolved.

Or . . . Life was going well until a trauma happened that made the client feel very vulnerable. No one protected them, no one comforted them. Then they remembered how good it felt when they ate chocolate chip cookies fresh out of the oven, and how much fun it was to eat pizza from the corner pizzeria—yet despite all the delicious food, deep down, they were still not comforted. And moreover, they felt shame about the way they were eating.

Another story told by Kathryn Sica, LMFT, CEDS, is about a client whose eating disorder started when attempting to deal with her parents' divorce. The client was angry with her mom, whom she blamed for the divorce. In order to express that anger, she would throw out the school lunch her mom packed for her every day. Not only did this give the client a sense of power, it also made her like the power of "not needing lunch" (denying she has needs).

Hence the journey begins down the rabbit hole to an eating disorder. The more stressful, uncomfortable, and overwhelming life becomes, the louder the eating disorder voice becomes. The voice promises to help individuals manage difficult situations, to help soothe them, to comfort them. All the individual has to do is follow the eating disorder's rules.

The problem is compounded by the society we live in, a society that supports the harmful messages of the eating disorder voice: Thinness and fitness are cherished. "Clean" diets are applauded. Food is not to be enjoyed, but feared.

In the beginning, most individuals don't realize they have a separate eating disorder self. Many times, this concept is introduced to them for the first time in treatment. They learn to distinguish between their healthy voice, who is open to recovery and freedom, and their eating disorder voice, who wants to keep them trapped in unhealthy behaviors. It is not uncommon, then, for clients to feel ambivalent about wanting recovery.

In my interview with Rebecca Clegg, LPC, CEDS-S, she shared

that "clients become frustrated with themselves, they emphatically express their desire for change and growth and freedom from their disorder; and yet they feel helpless. Even with these honest desires, they don't know why they don't follow through. The entrenched eating disorder identity leads to an enigma of equal parts: individuals want to get better and they also don't."

It is helpful for clients to learn that the battle against their eating disorder is an internal one. It is between their eating disorder self and their healthy self. Treatment providers need to help clients dialogue between their two selves and help the healthy self get back in control.

A helpful technique often used to begin this process is to teach the recovering individual how to turn down the volume of their eating disorder voice and amplify the voice of the healthy self. They have likely been listening to their eating disorder voice for so long, they would not recognize their healthy self even if it did speak up.

Research has shown that this "healthy self voice" can be helped by having clinicians teach their clients how to talk back and respond to the eating disorder voice. "When working with the voice, clinicians should aim to address both the content of the voice and how individuals relate and respond to it."[2]

The dialogue can begin by asking questions such as these:

- What can your healthy self tell your eating disorder self, who believes you will only be loved if you are thin?
- What can your healthy self tell your eating disorder self, who believes you are too weak and incompetent to handle your problems, and that food is your only friend?

As all the ways in which the eating disorder behaviors help the client cope with life are uncovered, the client is encouraged to ponder the question, "Is it worth it?"

If the eating disorder voice dictates, "You must exercise *x* amount of days for *x* amount of hours no matter what," are you really in control? Do you really want to deny yourself the enjoyment of eating all types of foods, and being able to eat at restaurants with your friends, so that you know the exact calories you consumed? Do you really want to risk tearing your esophagus each time you purge because you are unwilling to speak up to your boss? Do you really want to feel physically uncomfortable by routinely eating beyond fullness because you are afraid you will drown in your emotions if you sit with them?

The process of recovery involves continuous exploration, and questions and fears may arise. Here are some examples:

- If I eat more, will my body change?
- Will people comment on my body, whether it has changed or not?
- How will I face the world?
- How will I face my family or friends, my peers, or my coworkers?
- What else will make me feel unique or special?
- What can I do to be disciplined in my life?
- How will I learn to sit with my feelings?
- In what other ways will I punish myself?
- What will my life be like without all the lying?
- What will it be like to be honest or follow through on my word?
- What other interests in my life can I be this disciplined and structured with?
- What would it be like to be spontaneous and flexible in my life?
- Will I be out of control with food if I start eating or giving myself permission to eat what I want to eat?
- Is my life worth being "fat" to be "healthy"?
- Do I believe my team when I am told I could be happy and healthy?
- How has my eating disorder served me in my life?
- What would my life be like without my eating disorder?
- Who am I without my eating disorder?
- Am I enjoying the food I'm eating?
- Am I eating what I want, or what I believe I "should" be eating?
- What would I like to eat?
- What are my fears about eating what I would like?
- What would it be like to look at food for what it is, as opposed to having a number defining my choice?

- How would I feel if I didn't exercise for one or two days or more?
- Would my food choices be impacted if I didn't exercise?
- What would I want to do with my life that my eating disorder has held me back from doing?
- What will people think of me if I eat differently?
- What would it feel like to make myself a priority?
- What would it feel like to trust my own opinion?
- How would things change if I had different boundaries in my life?
- Do I care what people think about my actions around food?
- What would people think of me if I changed the conversation from something anti-food or movement-based?
- Can I trust my body to eat when I'm hungry and stop when I'm full?
- What would I tell somebody else to do in this same circumstance?

Saying Goodbye to the Eating Disorder Self

As you can imagine, letting go of an eating disorder is a complex and challenging process. In their book *Eating Disorders*, Reiff and Reiff use a metaphorical story ("The Helicopter Story") that illustrates the complexities of both the development of an eating disorder and the subsequent recovery process.[3] Imagine you are on an airplane and you do not know how to swim. You are not questioned if you know how to swim before going on the airplane. The plane crashes, and you are now in the ocean and grab a life preserver to survive. The life preserver is keeping you afloat. When you are in the ocean, you scan the skies and notice a helicopter flying above. After waving your hands, people from the helicopter see you. They say they will rescue you, but you have to let go of the life preserver. You are uncertain if they can rescue you. You do not want to give up the life preserver and question if you will be saved or experience hypothermia in the freezing water. The helicopter people become impatient and tell you that you must make a choice. Will you go with them, or wait for a lifeboat and take your life preserver with you? You hope that you can survive in the cold water without drowning or freezing to death.

The lifeboat is perfectly analogous to how treatment helps

individuals recover from an eating disorder. Instead of simply expecting them to let go of their eating disorder (their life preserver), you teach them how to swim first. To the individual, the eating disorder is what helped them survive. You cannot ask someone to let go of something without giving them something else (alternative tools) to hold on to. It is up to treatment professionals to help the client find other "life preserver" options that are not detrimental to their life and well-being.

It is because of the complexity of recovering from an eating disorder that it is imperative the treatment team be educated about eating disorders. Just like someone dealing with cancer would see an oncologist, or someone with kidney disease would see a nephrologist, eating disorders, no less life-altering, are best treated by a specialist. Making a transition from an existing therapist, dietitian, or doctor to one specialized in eating disorders may be difficult for the individual who has grown attached to their original providers. Explaining to the client that their original healthcare providers have served them well up to now, and that they now need the optimal support provided by specialists for their specific challenge, will help ease this transition.

As clients embark on their journey to recovery, their progress can happen in a nonlinear fashion. Some days will feel victorious, and other days a failure. An individual might agree in session about going from eating six grapes to twelve grapes, earnestly promising to try this before their next visit. But the second they walk out the door, their eating disorder voice throws their healthy self in the trunk and takes the wheel.

This tug-of-war can be confusing for the individual in treatment and for the treatment team. They can be dealing with an individual who wants to get recovered, and at the same time doesn't want to change their behaviors. The family often reacts negatively to these behaviors as well, feeling frustrated when a detour occurs. The family may view this detour as manipulation, lying, and attention-seeking behavior on the part of the recovering individual.

This is another reason why having an educated and highly specialized eating disorder–treatment team, that is also empathetic to the needs of someone with an eating disorder, is invaluable. A clinician or doctor who is unable to recognize these behaviors as usual roadblocks in eating disorder recovery might share the same views as the family.

They may also feel frustrated and become judgmental toward the person attempting to recover. This will absolutely get in the way of effective treatment and could damage the individual's chances for recovery.

An educated and specialized treatment team attuned to the needs of people with eating disorders can also educate the family to anticipate and understand such behaviors. Where they might feel frustrated, a specialist can explain that a relapse or setback only proves how strong the eating disorder voice is, and how treatment and interventions can be appropriately adjusted.

Naturally, as one begins to question their disordered eating behaviors and consider recovery, they start questioning what life will look like without their eating disorder. They can become so scared of this unknown future that sometimes they would rather surrender to the disorder. It feels safer to live a small life of known restriction and limitation than a larger, unknown life of eating what they like, keeping food down, and being recovered.

Hence, the recovery process is one of trial and error. Every lapse, relapse, or misstep is an opportunity for growth and learning. Asking clients what happened that led them on a detour or created a misstep can help identify triggers. Once triggers are identified, they can be taught how to cope with them in a more positive way. It is hard to recognize such patterns, and even more difficult to change them, but with every attempt, the recovering individual becomes stronger in their fight for recovery.

Per my colleague, Kathryn Sica, "We want our clients to step out onto the battlefield and fight their eating disorder. Whether they win or lose the battle, they will learn something each time they step onto the battlefield, and will eventually win the war."

Another valuable tool used in recovery is having the client write a letter to their body and to their eating disorder. Perhaps this can be done in the beginning of treatment, considering what you will want to say to your body later on, praising it for not failing you during this time. You might simply acknowledge all your body allows you to do, like carry groceries or a backpack, hug and kiss your loved ones, walk in nature. You might appreciate your body's attunement and how it has supported you through life, letting you know when you are hungry or cold or hurt. Writing a letter to your eating disorder can clarify how it has served you, and what it has at the same time taken away from you.

As my colleague, Rebecca Clegg, shared with me, "The treatment team can help the individual by highlighting the part that wants to get better, the part that wants a life worth living. Begin by asking that part to show up. What would the person who decided to come to treatment, the one who did the research and is investing in treatment, the part that wants to get better . . . what would that person say?"

It is up to treatment professionals to help individuals in recovery find compassion for themselves, something they have likely not had for many years, if at all ever. Compassion in their journey, compassion in their struggles, compassion in their frustrations, and compassion for their body and the transitions it is going through.

Eating disorders often evolve as a maladaptive coping skill to get through a life challenge. With appropriate treatment, clients learn to explore the purpose of their eating disorder self. They learn that their eating disorder self can be a nondominant part of who they are, and that they don't have to engage in its prescribed behaviors. Those behaviors were needed when they lacked other skills to help them survive the difficult parts of life. When their tool chest is full, and they are experienced in utilizing its contents, the eating disorder will ultimately be put out of a job. Now the client's job becomes creating a more authentic version of themselves who is willing to live a full life. Pointing out that it is the client's healthy self that has them show up for treatment sessions, and has them be motivated for change, begins to turn the tides in their ability to recognize that their eating disorder life preserver is not the only way to survive.

Chapter 12 Notes

1. Carolyn Costin and Gwen Grabb, *8 Keys to Recovery from an Eating Disorder: Effective Strategies from Therapeutic Practice and Personal Experience* (New York: W. W. Norton & Company, Inc., 2012).

2. N. Scott, T. L. Hanstock, and C. Thornton, "Dysfunctional self-talk associated with eating disorder severity and symptomatology," *Journal of Eating Disorders* 2, no. 14 (May 2014), doi: 10.1186/2050-2974-2-14.

3. Dan Reiff and Kathleen Reiff, *Eating Disorders: Nutrition Therapy in the Recovery Process* (Alphen aan den Rijn, Netherlands: Aspen Publishers, 1992), 3–4.

CHAPTER 13

DIVIDE AND CONQUER: MEET YOUR TEAM

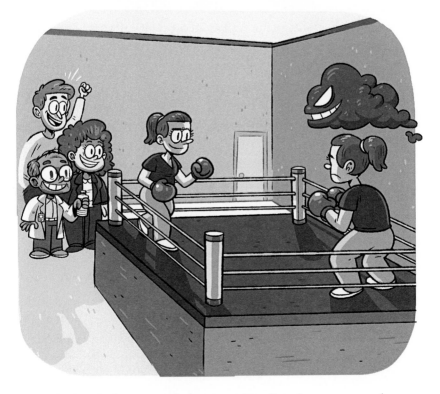

In the battle for survival that is eating disorder recovery, the treatment team is the force that supports the fight. This army is only as strong as each individual member's ability to perform their roles and work with one another effectively.

The treatment team must collaborate on the emotional, physiological, and behavioral elements involved in treating the client with an eating disorder. This calls for team members to contribute their individualized specialty and expertise in supporting, educating, and caring for the recovering client. It is imperative that all team members understand this collaboration to ensure that they all "stay in their lane" in regard to performing their own valuable roles, while also allowing their counterparts to do the same.

In this sense, they must collaboratively divide and conquer.

It is a process to create an effective treatment team. Often, clients do not approach an eating disorder specialist for treatment and/or are not provided with the opportunity to create their own team from scratch. It is more common for there to be an existing team already in place, which might include preexisting relationships with a mental health provider, physician, pediatrician, registered dietitian, and psychiatrist. As a dietitian specializing in eating disorders, I often have clients who already have sought out and received help from other professionals they trust. However, these other health professionals may be neither educated in nor specialize in eating disorders in the first place. As you can imagine, this creates an entirely different set of issues for us all to tackle.

It is important to discuss the potential conflicts that can arise from such situations. Although this can be a difficult and awkward discussion to have, the ultimate goal is to provide the best care for the client. It is not uncommon for clinicians not trained in eating disorders to be uncomfortable dealing with such cases. Their lack of expertise may cause the clinician to make statements that may actually stall the client's recovery. The unfortunate truth is that schools offer little, if any, eating disorder training. Professionals often receive their training through working in treatment centers, obtaining supervision, attending conferences, or by their own "lived experience." It is the responsibility of the clinician to know their limits, and recognize when the client's situation is out of their realm of expertise.

It is imperative to appropriately support the client when there is a need to change or make additions to the client's treatment team. Clients need to feel they still have control and their input matters. It is important that they not feel abandoned by previous health providers, but rather respected enough to be given specialized care. We usually accomplish this goal by tapering down visits with the existing clinician, and increasing visits with the new registered dietitian and/or mental health provider.

Every person in recovery has their own individual needs. Therefore, the makeup of the treatment team should be individualized, and not "cookie cutter." The person's diagnoses, physical needs, location logistics, finances, and other contributing factors should be considered when choosing the professionals on their treatment team. The most common recommendation, supported by research, is to at the minimum have a medical doctor, individual therapist, and registered dietitian on the team. Of course, all the team members need to be educated in or specialize in eating disorders.[1]

The registered dietitian's role is to educate the client on how their eating disorder is impacting their body and overall well-being. This can be done by complementing what the physician may have already discussed with the client in reviewing lab results, vital signs, and bone density tests. In addition, the dietitian can specifically address the downside and impact of starvation, purging, binging, compulsively exercising, laxative abuse, or any other disordered behavior the client may be engaging in.

The dietitian provides the client with facts in order to dispel any myths about food. The dietitian will support the client in the often-times frightening process of renourishing themselves, healing body image, and providing self-care. This is done by teaching the client how to connect to their body when they are going through nutritional rehabilitation. Questions such as what different foods feel like on their lips, how food tastes, and how food feels in their body can help the client become aware of all the properties of food (not just their calorie content, for example) and become attuned to their bodily sensations.

Ultimately, the dietitian will help the client see the impact of their negative food and body thoughts on their life, and help to bring perspective and compassion back into the client's life. Because clients often see their registered dietitian more frequently than their physician, the dietitian's role becomes a very important and impactful one.

While the dietitian and physician's focus is on healing the physical and nutritional rehabilitation of the person recovering from an eating disorder, the therapist's focus is on the emotional recovery. As the previous chapter explored, eating disorders are often adaptive coping mechanisms, and it is the role of the therapist to explore this with the recovering individual. The therapist will help the client dig deep to get to the crux of the role the eating disorder has played in their life.

The areas most therapists explore typically involve temperament, the familial or societal messages clients have been given about food, their body and appearance, and how that is related to self-worth and self-love. In order to discover where the drive for thinness, for example, may come from, therapists consider the impact of any trauma, comorbid mental health diagnoses, invalidating environments and support systems, or a history of bullying. Conversely, the client may be overeating to suppress feelings or to develop a protective barrier to keep people at a distance. Identifying what function the eating disorder plays for the client is very helpful.

In working toward recovery, the therapist's role is to help the client rewrite these narratives, to feel their feelings, and to challenge their thoughts. It is also to build a new concept of how to integrate their disorder and explore their healthy self, which will heal their eating disorder self.[2] The therapist helps the recovering individual understand the emotional underpinnings of their disorder, as well as conceptualize a future without it. Together they explore what it would be like to be sufficient, to have a career, to have insight into what they want in their life, and how to shift from a place of obsession with body dissatisfaction to a place of body satisfaction or body tolerance.[3]

A part of the treatment team also includes the patient's family. Gaining the support of loved ones can be difficult, but an unequivocally important part of treatment. It is very helpful for family members to be in their own therapy as well. This not only supports the identified patient, but also helps the family explore their own relationship with food and their bodies. Family therapy also assists the client's support system to not blame themselves for their loved one's disorder, and teaches them effective communication skills. If unable to afford a therapist, there are many support groups and online resources available for family members.

An essential component of collaboration among team members is having a signed consent. A signed consent technically gives permission to team members to discuss applicable client information with each other. Due to HIPPA (Health Insurance Portability and Accountability

Act) laws, it is unethical for any mental health or medical professional to discuss the private health information of a client without such a consent (if they are over eighteen years of age). The ability to seamlessly communicate with each other allows all the team members access to life situations that may be impacting the client, leading to more cohesive treatment. This communication is especially important for clients who may also have coexisting challenges, such as substance abuse.

Each of these professionals would be easily accessible in a perfect world. The reality, however, is that the ability to pay for and obtain all such services is not possible for all clients. It is not uncommon, then, for a professional to wear many hats, if that is what the client needs. There is no hard and fast rule, for example, that says a dietitian cannot also discuss with a client the emotional impact of food and body image. As a treatment provider, if you do find yourself in such a situation, however, it is your responsibility to educate yourself to ensure you are providing accurate, safe, and helpful information. This can be done by consulting with an expert, obtaining supervision, and/or attending specialized training sessions.

When the expertise of all these professionals merges in the appropriate way, it enhances the recovering individual's ability to heal mind, body, and soul. This brings us to a core value that everyone involved in the treatment team must have: empathic collaboration. A provider who agrees to treat an individual with an eating disorder needs to have this trait in order to effectively and compassionately treat the individual.

Treatment team members must examine themselves, their motivations, and their own relationship with food, body, and diet culture. Are the client's needs and welfare the priority? Are decisions made in the best interest of the client? Does the clinician have any judgment about weight that may lead to weight stigmatization? The clinician's perception will impact all recommendations they make. For example, does the clinician believe the individual can be recovered? It is critical for treatment providers to know that people can completely get over their eating disorder and become recovered. If they have a warped relationship with their bodies, food, or movement, then they can end up colluding with the client's disease. It is therefore imperative for each team member to resolve any such issues, so that they can treat clients with a weight-neutral and inclusive approach. Approaching recovering individuals with nonjudgment, compassion, and kindness will help them feel supported as they trudge the long and challenging road to recovery.

Treatment team empathy increases the client's openness to treatment and recovery. Clients will be more open to exploring their most harmful and negative thoughts about themselves and the world, and be more engaged in recovery, if they feel they will not be ridiculed or judged. Let's face it, we are all more likely to take positive action when we trust the person suggesting the action will not harm or judge us. Clients are more likely to be invested in their treatment if they feel empathy from their team, and this level of engagement is crucial for treatment success.

Treatment requires so much of clients, emotionally, physically, and mentally. Their connection with the treatment team allows them to navigate recovery with less fear. We ask clients to relinquish their safety blankets, and trust that we will give them something more fulfilling, joyous, and helpful back. Activities like creating hope collages for the future, creating healing art, teaching the joy of food and cooking, letting go of clothes that no longer fit, restoring weight, being open to self-care, and learning to recognize and use their own voice are beautifully transformative, but they cannot happen without treatment team empathy creating a safe space for the recovering individual to engage.

Treatment team members can learn more about empathy by educating themselves about eating disorders from an emotional, psychological, biological, and social perspective. I advise all eating disorder professionals to attend supervision meetings. Such meetings provide support and insight from other professionals in the field. Attending local or national conferences is also a great way to increase one's knowledge and expertise. These venues also provide an opportunity for networking with other professionals who can be great resources in the field. Some examples of such organizations are the Academy for Eating Disorders (AED), International Association of Eating Disorders Professionals (IAEDP), and the National Eating Disorders Association (NEDA).

The knowledge and understanding of eating disorders gained from the above-mentioned resources can be used to create treatment dream teams. These are teams that prioritize the client; provide nonjudgmental, supportive, and compassionate care; and empower and embolden clients to fight for their recovery.

Any professional who engages with children, teens, or adults struggling with or recovering from eating disorders has an incredible opportunity to create world-shifting change in the lives of others and in the reduction of eating disorders. This change can result from early diagnosis, more effective and well-rounded treatment, increased awareness and recovery rates, and decreased rates of eating disorder–related deaths. It all starts with an informed treatment team who has empathy. That one small but invaluable trait opens the door to learning, education, awareness, coordination, understanding, support, freedom, and life.

Chapter 13 Notes

1. K. Halimi, "Salient components of a comprehensive service for eating disorders," *World Psychiatry* 8, no. 3 (October 2009): 150–155.

2. Carolyn Costin and Gwen Grabb, *8 Keys to Recovery from an Eating Disorder: Effective Strategies from Therapeutic Practice and Personal Experience* (New York: W. W. Norton & Company, Inc., 2012), 37–61.

3. Carolyn Costin and Gwen Grabb, *8 Keys to Recovery*, 93–122.

ACKNOWLEDGMENTS

This book could not have happened without an amazing team: Justin Spizman, my book architect; Margot Rittenhouse, my ghostwriter; Austin Baechle, my illustrator; and the entire team at BookLogix. I wanted to thank the following people, who are more than colleagues to me. I am fortunate to have them as friends and expert contributors to the book: Carolyn Costin, Kevin Wandler, Pam Carlton, Lesley Williams, Edward Tyson, Becca Clegg, and Kathy Sica.

The following individuals have been wonderful expert reviewers, valued colleagues, and friends: Jill Sechi, Anna Lutz, Stephanie Brooks, Marci Evans, Ralph Carson, Leslie Schilling, Lesley Kaplan, Jennifer Gaudiani, Nancy King, Pam Kelle, Kathy Cortese, Reba Sloan, Francie White, Diana Lipson-Burge, Buck Runyan, and Ovidio Bermudez.

A special thank-you to Shazi Shabatian and Kevin Wandler for their support, patience, expertise, friendship, and being my backup set of eyes. I also wanted to thank my colleague and friend Andrew Sage Mendez-McLeish for reviewing and editing language respecting gender. Thank you, Louise Stanger, for your ongoing support and encouragement.

Lastly, thank you to my family for their ongoing love: my mother, who is my cheerleader; my dad, who always was proud of my hard work and dedication for anything I put my mind to; my husband, Mike, for his patience and clever ideas; and my puppies Madison and Hudson, who have been extremely patient and loving with me.

ABOUT THE AUTHOR

Robyn L. Goldberg, RDN, CEDRD-S, began her career at Cedars-Sinai Medical Center in Los Angeles as the in-patient dietitian in the department of cardiology. Over the last twenty-three years, she has developed her own private practice in Beverly Hills, California, where she specializes in medical conditions, disordered eating, eating disorders, Health at Every Size, pre-pregnancy nutrition, and people in recovery. Robyn is a Certified Eating Disorders Registered Dietitian and Supervisor from IAEDP and a Certified Intuitive Eating Counselor. For the last eight years Robyn was the nutrition counselor for an outpatient eating disorder program, and led eating disorder and body image groups at various sober livings in Los Angeles. She is a contributing author and nationally known registered dietitian nutritionist. She has been quoted in the *New York Times*, the *Huffington Post*, *The Fix*, *Shape* magazine, *Fitness*, *Oxygen*, *Pilates Style*, *Diabetes Forecast*, *BH Weekly*, and *Life & Style*. She has been on national television as the eating disorder expert on *The Insider*.

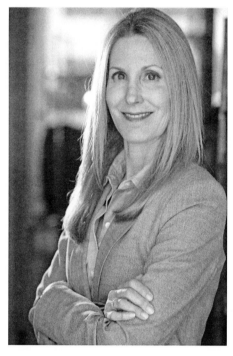